CH00705114

OUR HOSPITAL

The Royal United Hospital, Bath

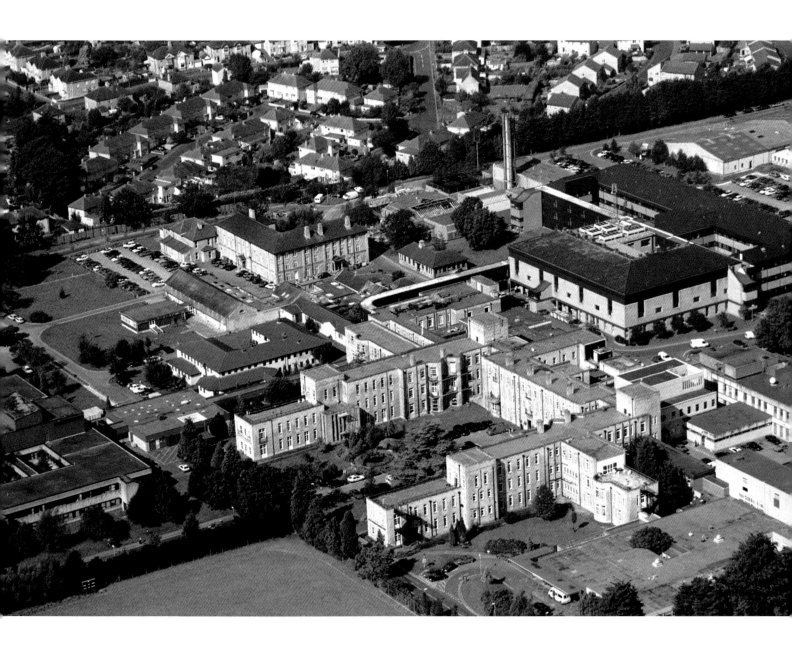

OUR HOSPITAL

The Royal United Hospital, Bath

Tim Craft

*All proceeds from sales of this book go to the
hospital's charitable fund*

Published on behalf of the Royal United Hospital, Bath
by BIOS Scientific Publishers Ltd, Oxford, UK

© BIOS Scientific Publishers Ltd, 1998

First published 1998

All rights reserved. No part of this book may be reproduced
or transmitted, in any form or by any means, without permission.

A CIP catalogue record for this book is available from the British Library.

ISBN 1 85996 002 2

BIOS Scientific Publishers Ltd
9 Newtec Place, Magdalen Road, Oxford OX4 1RE, UK
Tel. 01865 726286 Fax 01865 246823

Images scanned by Dr Mike Scott

Designed by Design/Section, Frome

Printed and bound by Butler & Tanner Ltd, Frome and London

"RUH 2001 is our vision for the Royal United Hospital. It is a vision that has been developed by our clinical staff together with the General Practitioners and patients that we serve. It is a vision that gives us confidence that we will be able to continue to provide the best possible care for our patients. With the commencement of the site redevelopment the vision is becoming a reality."

Gerald Chown, Chairman

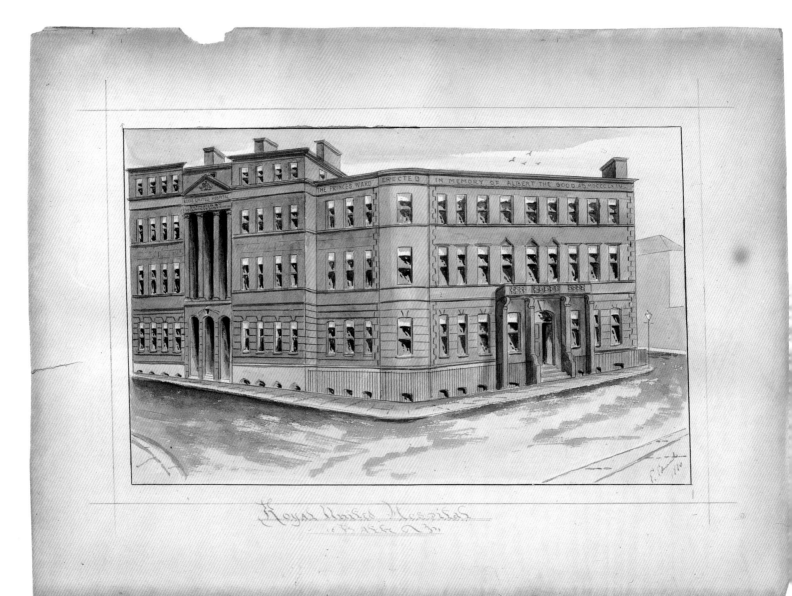

6

History in the making

In the early part of the eighteenth century the popularity of Bath as a health resort grew rapidly based upon the perceived benefits of the spa waters. With urban development came increasing poverty and public health problems. In this way Bath was no different from any other expanding city, and it was apparent that the less well-off populations of Bath required access to some form of health care. To this end the Bath Pauper Trust was established in 1747 and a dispensary opened in Wood Street. The origins of the Royal United Hospital can be traced back to this humble beginning. Initially, the Dispensary offered advice and treatment to patients on an outpatient basis only but as the need for inpatient facilities grew it was extended and in 1792 became known as the Bath City Infirmary and Dispensary.

By the second half of the eighteenth century construction work on many of Bath's now famous architectural landmarks, such as the Royal Crescent, The Circus, The Parade, and Pulteney Bridge, was well underway. Just as today, such work inevitably resulted in a number of accidents and casualties. In 1788 a private house was converted and the Casualty Hospital opened specifically to care for the victims of such accidents. For the next 35 years health care for the citizens of Bath continued to be provided by these two institutions; the Bath City Infirmary and Dispensary and the Casualty Hospital.

(Left) The original Royal United Hospital and Albert Wing in Beau Street.

(Below) The beautiful Pulteney Bridge, one of Bath's many famous architectural landmarks.

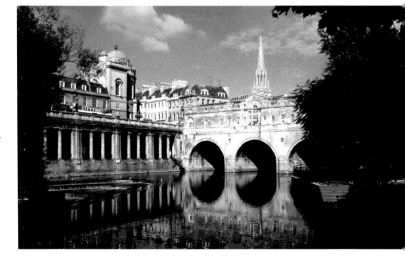

By the early 1820s it was obvious that the two hospitals duplicated services in a number of areas and it seemed mutually beneficial that they merge. After a period of consultation it was agreed that a new hospital should be built in what is now Beau Street. The foundation stone was laid in 1824 and 2 years later the Bath United Hospital opened to patients.

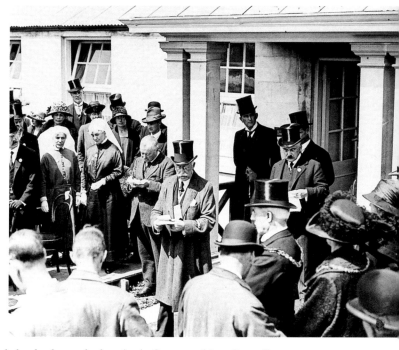

The hospital continued to treat ever increasing numbers of patients and by 1860 there was a desperate need for additional inpatient accommodation. In 1861 Prince Albert, Consort to Queen Victoria, died from typhoid fever and it was agreed that a new wing for the hospital should be commissioned as a memorial to the Prince. On 23 May 1864, amid a great deal of pomp and circumstance and to the sound of the Abbey bells a procession moved slowly through the city before reaching Beau Street. The foundation stone to the Albert Wing was then laid and construction commenced on an extension to the hospital. Following the completion of the extension and the dedication of its wards to Prince Albert, Queen Victoria announced that she would be pleased to allow the hospital thereafter to be known as the Royal United Hospital, Bath.

For many years the position of the hospital remained broadly unchanged, close to the physical centre of the city and caring for the people of Bath and the surrounding towns and villages.

It was not until the First World War that a hospital was established in Combe Park, the current site of the RUH. In 1916 the Bath War Hospital was opened with 500 beds to provide for the treatment of wounded soldiers. This hospital, which included an X-ray department, operating theatres and physiotherapy facilities, was not closed until 1929. Meanwhile, on an adjacent site at Combe Park the Forbes Fraser Hospital was opened in 1924 as a private hospital. In the same year the Children's Orthopaedic Hospital was also opened and 12 months later the number of beds was more than tripled. This hospital later became the Bath and Wessex Orthopaedic Hospital.

With medical advances demanding more space and more patients requiring treatment, the hospital had

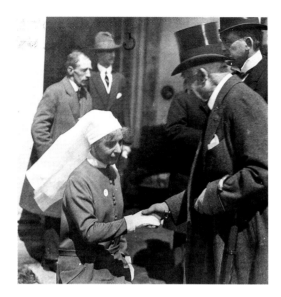

(Above and left) The opening ceremony of the Combe Park Forbes Fraser Hospital by HRH The Duke of Connaught, 16 May 1924.

outgrown its site in Beau Street by the late 1920s. Despite the poor financial climate an appeal was commenced in the 1930s to raise funds so the hospital could move to its current site in Combe Park. The city of Bath rose to the challenge and the necessary funds were acquired for the commencement of the construction of what is now RUH South. As many patients as possible were discharged home and on 11 December 1932 the Royal United Hospital finally moved from its site in Beau Street to the new hospital in Combe Park.

At that time the RUH had for neighbours the closed War Hospital, the Forbes Fraser Hospital, and The Bath and Wessex Children's Orthopaedic Hospital.

Less than 7 years after the move to Combe Park war broke out again and in 1940 Manor House and adjacent grounds were requisitioned for use as a military hospital. For a while this was run by American forces and when they left at the end of the second World War the remaining hospital was known as the Manor Hospital. At the time of the birth of the National Health Service in 1948, the site at Combe Park was home to four quite separate hospitals.

A number of smaller building projects continued over the following years and in 1959 the Ear, Nose and Throat Hospital in Marlborough Buildings closed and moved to Combe Park. By 1970 the Manor Hospital had been retitled RUH (North) and in 1973 the Bath Eye Infirmary also moved to the RUH site. In 1978 building work was started on the Princess Anne Wing and in 1981 HRH Princess Anne opened that part of the hospital which currently houses maternity services. In 1993 the New Ward Block was opened together with a suite of operating theatres and the Intensive Therapy and Coronary Care Units.

Exactly 250 years after the opening of the first hospital to which it can trace its origins, the Royal United Hospital, Bath is entering perhaps the most exciting phase of its physical development. Our hospital has constantly changed and evolved in response to the needs of the patients it serves. As we enter the next century, we do so with the confidence that our vision for the hospital following the redevelopment (RUH 2001) offers the best opportunity for us all to ensure that the RUH continues to offer the very highest standards of care to all its patients.

For the future...

For some years it has been apparent that the linking together of so many disparate buildings at the RUH does not produce a very efficient or user-friendly site for a thriving hospital. There are many long corridors, maintenance and heating costs are high (especially of the older buildings), and the RUH lacks a central focus. There are a number of ways in to the hospital but no obvious main entrance that all patients and visitors can find their way to and from. Furthermore, there have been clinical advances that render the current hospital less than ideal as an environment in which to care for the sick. More and more treatments or procedures are carried out on an outpatient or short stay basis, whilst those who are admitted to the hospital as inpatients tend to require increasingly complex investigations and management.

With these patient-focused concerns in mind it was decided to bid for funding to redevelop certain aspects of the hospital. Doctors, nurses, and other healthcare workers formed small groups to address the needs of their own clinical areas. Architects were commissioned and met with the various groups and the plans for RUH 2001 started to take shape. The advice of Bath and North East Somerset Council was sought and colleagues in general practice and the neighbouring community hospitals were consulted. Eventually a more compact, more flexible design for the hospital was agreed upon and, despite a fiercely competitive climate in which to try to win public funds, to everyone's delight the NHS approved our plans for the redevelopment of the Royal United Hospital, Bath.

We believe that the new look RUH should include:

- integrated services for many specialties where patients will receive inpatient and outpatient treatment in the same location from the same group of specialist staff;
- a new centralised children's unit which will address the problems resulting from the current facilities being spread around the site;
- an assessment unit for the elderly, improving services for this group of patients;
- a new specialist breast care unit where a multidisciplinary group of professionals will work side by side to provide the most effective assessment and treatment for breast disease;
- state of the art facilities for diagnosing illness in an environment which is modern, efficient, and caring;
- improved accident and emergency facilities;
- a purpose-built day surgery unit;
- modernised hospital wards.

As well as bringing hospital services closer together, the redevelopment will provide a new main entrance and a central focus to the RUH, resulting in a much easier environment in which to be a patient, a visitor, or indeed, a member of staff.

A caring community

The Royal United Hospital is the acute district general hospital for a population of around 450 000 people. Approximately 80 000 live in the city of Bath but the majority live in the market towns and villages that lie around Bath in Wiltshire, Avon, and North East Somerset.

Many of the market towns have their own community hospitals with whom the RUH works closely. Consultant staff travel to these hospitals to undertake outpatient clinics and see patients referred by their General Practitioner. Some patients are discharged from the RUH to a bed in their community hospital before being well enough to go home completely, and at some of the hospitals surgeons from the RUH perform operations under local anaesthesia. Many women deliver their babies in their local community hospital, whilst the acute hospital backup for those mothers or babies who require more acute care is provided at the RUH. With the advent of new technologies such as telemedicine it will be possible for a

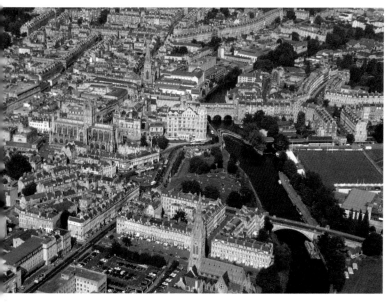

doctor seeing a patient in a community hospital to seek an immediate specialist opinion from the RUH of, for instance, a skin rash or an X-ray. As we enter the next century the RUH will continue to develop its relationship with the community hospitals around it.

The RUH is one of the largest employers in Bath. It is the place of work for around 2200 people. Everyone at the hospital has been involved in some way with RUH 2001 and everyone will share in the sense of pride when the redevelopment is complete. The RUH exists for us all whether we are patients, relatives of patients, people who might one day be patients, or members of staff at the hospital. The Royal United Hospital, Bath is *Our Hospital*.

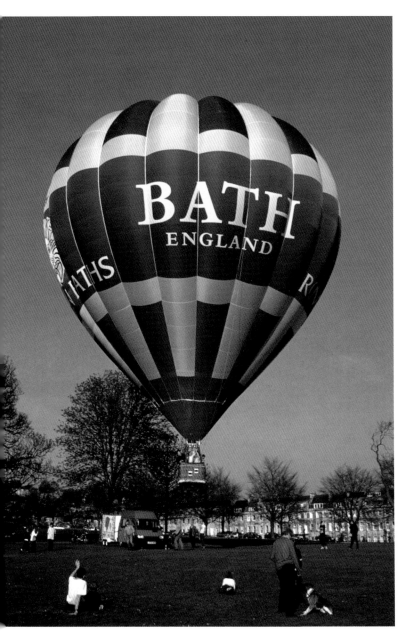

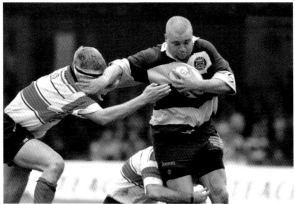

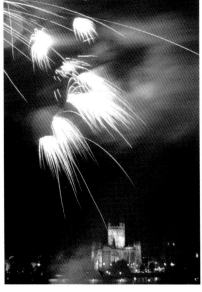

The RUH also provides the acute hospital back up for all the cultural, sporting, and social events that take place in and around the city.

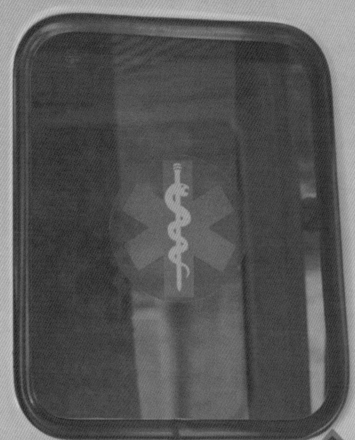

ANCE

612
TO OPEN

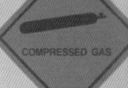
COMPRESSED GAS
2

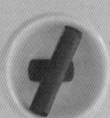

ENCY

Master

Accident & Emergency

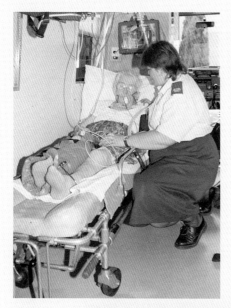

For many patients A&E is the front door to the hospital. The majority of patients who are admitted to the RUH as emergencies are first seen in this department. Each year 45 000 new patients attend A&E, 20% of whom are children and 17% of whom are over the age of 75 years. Of these new patients 30% are admitted to the hospital. The A&E Department is of course open 24 hours a day, 365 days of the year for patients that require emergency treatment.

Bath has a large number of towns around it with their own community hospitals where the less unwell often attend for emergency treatment. This means that those patients who come to the RUH tend to be more severely unwell than in the average A&E Department. This is reflected in the fact that the RUH has the highest percentage of patients attending the A&E Department by ambulance than any other similar department in the country.

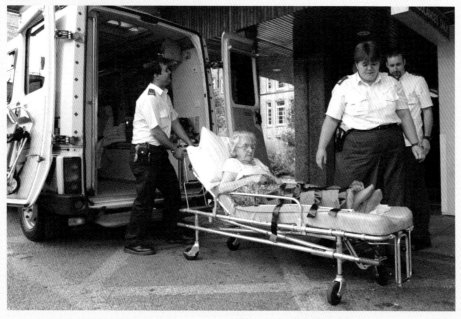

Patients arriving by ambulance often have critical medical or surgical illnesses requiring emergency treatment or may have suffered severe trauma in accidents. As with the rest of the hospital, the patient population served by the A&E Department is approximately 450 000 and they may live as far as 25 miles away.

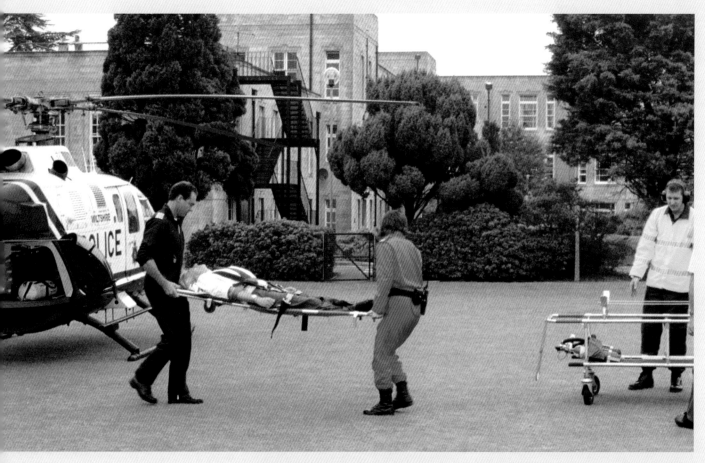

Because our patients tend to be more unwell and because distances travelled may be large, a significant number of patients arrive at the RUH by air ambulance. The helicopter is the Wiltshire police helicopter which is used 65% of the time for police duties and 35% of the time as an ambulance. Wiltshire ambulance service train and provide a paramedic for every medical callout the helicopter attends. The helicopter is especially useful for transporting victims of major trauma to the hospital quickly and lands on the edge of the cricket pitch just outside the A&E Department. Sometimes the air ambulance may take a team of doctors from A&E or Intensive Care to the scene of a road traffic accident before air lifting victims back to the RUH.

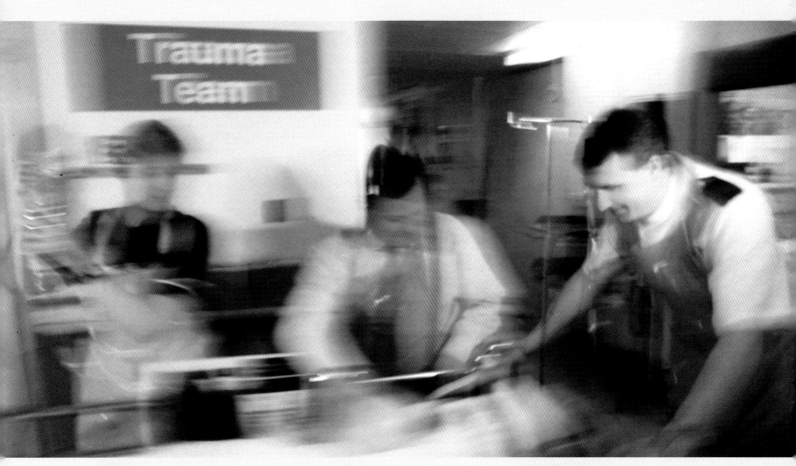

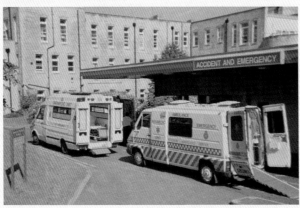

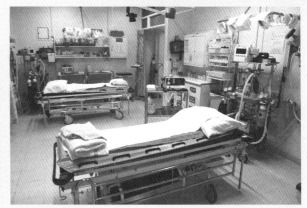

Once in the department, patients are seen and treated by a multidisciplinary team of healthcare workers. The composition of the team varies according to the needs of the patient so that the most appropriate care may be given. For example, a patient who has suffered a heart attack may be admitted by a medical team and be attended by the cardiac nurse practitioner who administers "clot-busting" drugs immediately after arrival. Some of the local GPs also work in the department as Clinical Assistants, thus helping to bridge the gap between General Practice and hospital care. The hospital's specialists may be called to the department to advise on the treatment of patients with particular illnesses.

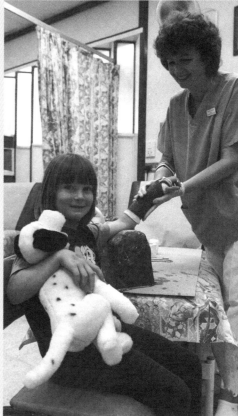

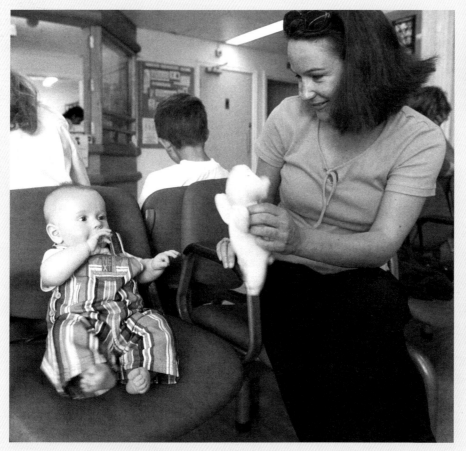

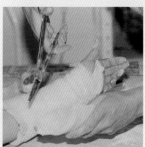

Many of the patients who attend the department have fractures that require stabilising with a plaster. Over 12 000 plasters are applied each year to patients at the RUH. Children often have light weight coloured plasters fitted.

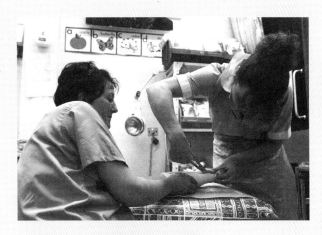

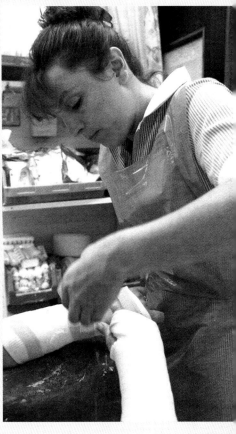

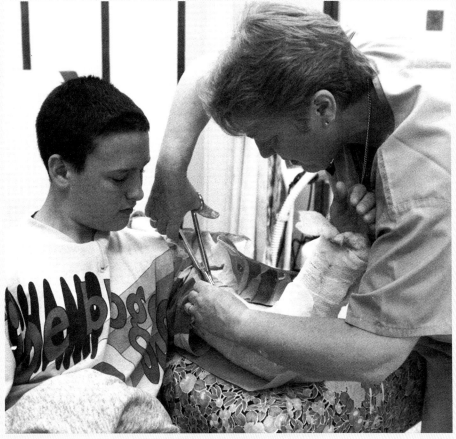

The Staff

The RUH is one of the largest employers in Bath. Indeed, the greatest investment we make is in our staff. The hospital is committed to developing all its staff to enable them to maximise their potential as individuals. The greatest strength of the RUH, however, comes from the way individuals work together in teams to deliver state-of-the-art medical care that focuses on each patient's needs. In this book we show just a few of the hospital's staff, in no particular order, doing what they do best; caring for patients.

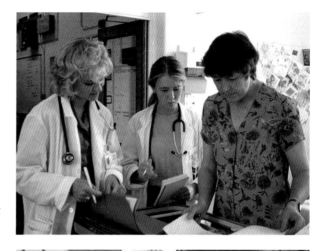

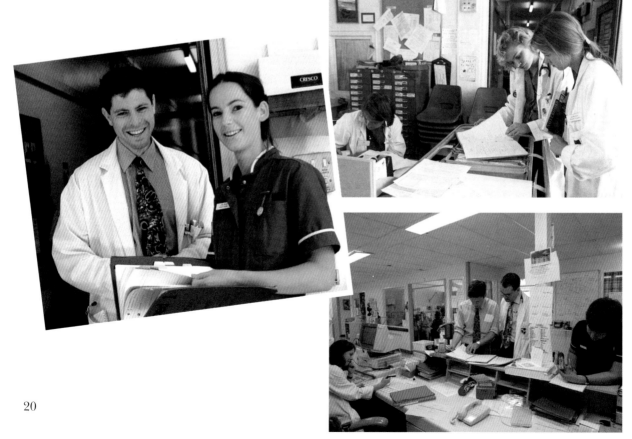

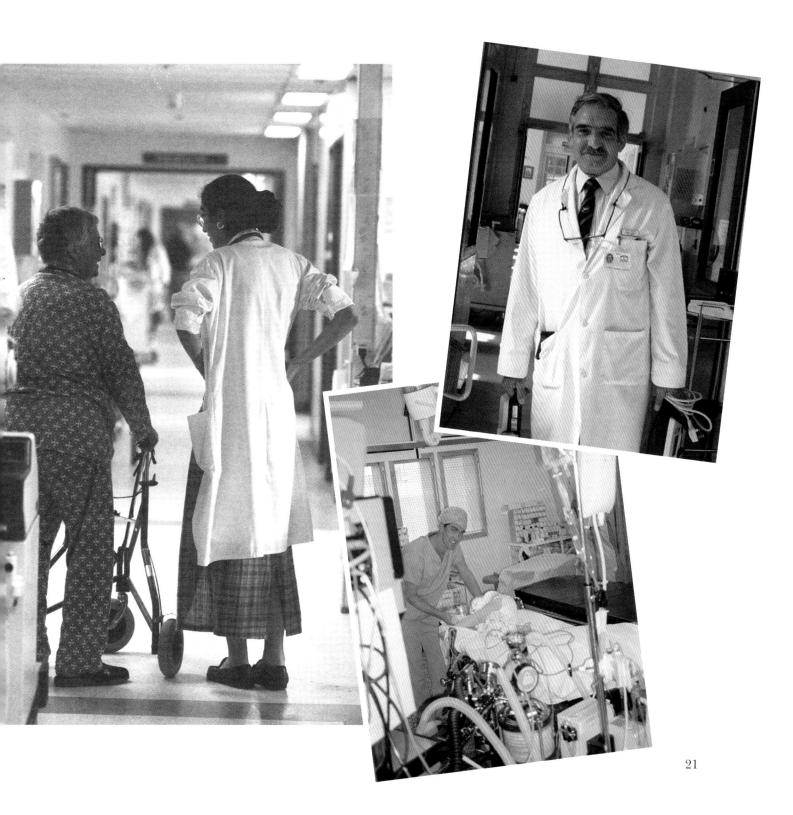

21

Pacemakers

Pacemakers are small implantable devices that are able to stimulate a heart beat with a small electrical signal. Pacemakers are able to sense when the heart is beating too slowly and then produce a stimulus appropriately. Some pacemakers are able to mimic heart function totally, certain models even have the ability to detect movement and so speed up the heart during exercise. Others are able to control very fast heart rates as well as stimulate the heart when the rate is too slow.

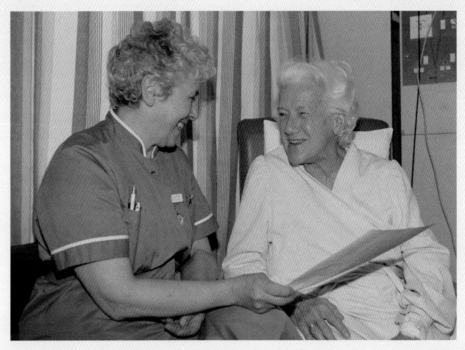

Mrs Hilda Guy is an 87 year old lady who was suffering blackouts caused by her heart beating too slowly. She was admitted to the RUH to have a pacemaker fitted.

Around 250 patients per year have a permanent pacemaker fitted at the RUH. The pacemaker itself costs between £1000 and £4000 and usually takes about an hour to insert. The unit is fitted beneath the skin below the collar bone under local anaesthesia.

A pacemaker may be as small as a 50 pence piece and may weigh as little as 23 grams (equivalent to the weight of two 50 pence pieces).

Patients usually stay one night in hospital following insertion of the device. They are then seen in the Out Patient Clinic once or twice a year to ensure that the pacemaker continues to function correctly. These checks are made externally and take just a few minutes. Pacemakers generally last between 7 and 10 years before the battery runs out.

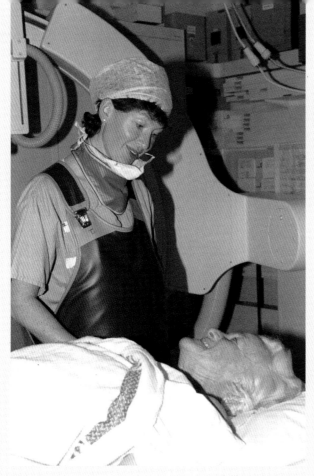

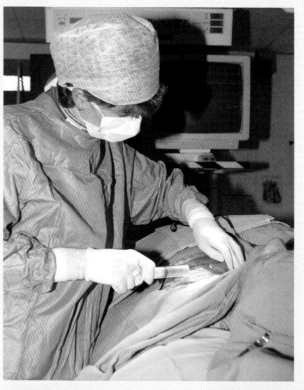

(Above) Mrs Guy was then positioned on a special operating table which allows an X-ray camera and TV screen to be used during the operation.

(Above right) The site where the device was to be fitted was then made numb with local anaesthetic before the pacemaker was implanted.

(Right) Following this the X-ray camera was used to observe the correct placement of the device.

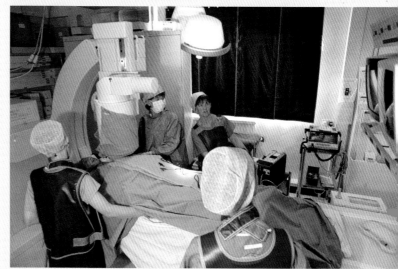

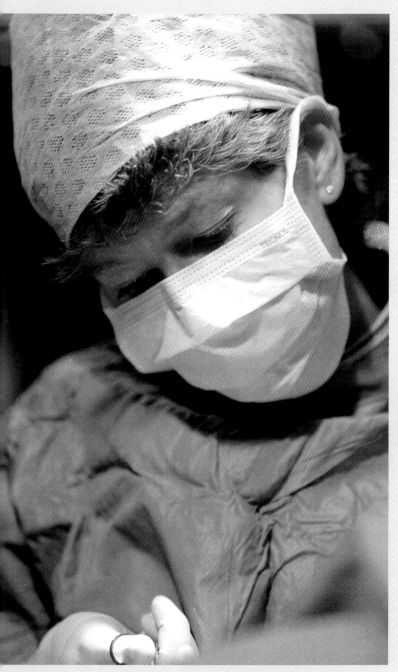

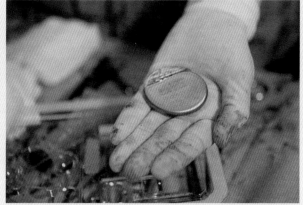

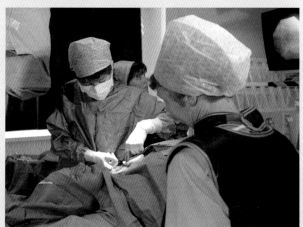

(Top right) The pacemaker
itself just prior to being inserted
beneath Mrs Guy's skin (above
and left).

(Right) A dressing was applied
after the incision had been
stitched closed. Throughout
the whole procedure Mrs Guy
was awake and able to talk to
her team.

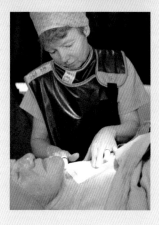

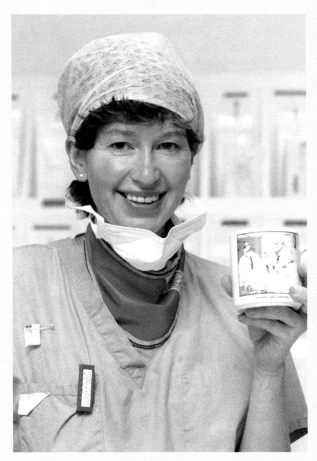

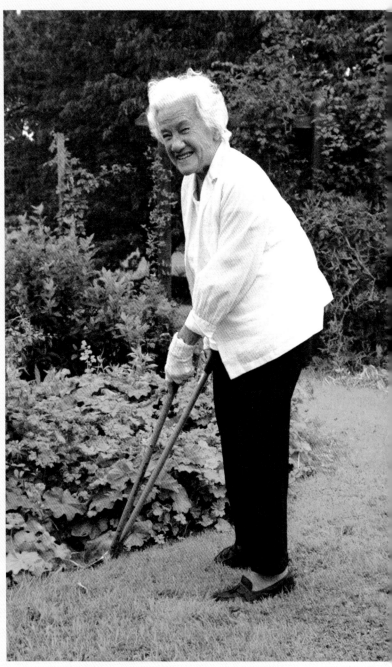

(Above) Dr Ruth Grabham is a General Practitioner in Bath who works part time in the Department of Cardiology as a Clinical Assistant. She has developed considerable expertise in the insertion of cardiac pacemakers and is representative of the close working relationship between doctors at the RUH and General Practitioners.

(Right) Since insertion of the pacemaker Mrs Guy has had no further blackouts and has been able to return to looking after her magnificent garden.

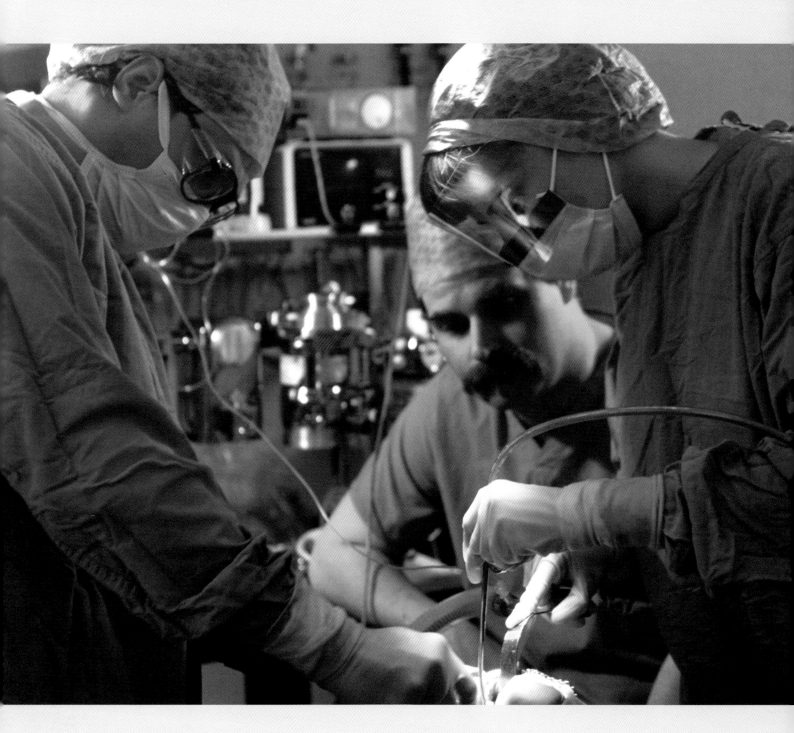

Maxillofacial Surgery

The Department of Oral and Maxillofacial Surgery at the RUH provides a variety of services including salivary gland surgery, care of patients with facial trauma, and surgical removal of teeth too difficult to be extracted by dental practitioners. The department also provides an integrated head and neck cancer service with colleagues in Ear, Nose and Throat. The Orthodontic Department, who specialise in re-aligning poorly positioned teeth, accept referrals for particularly difficult orthodontic problems. Outpatient clinics are undertaken in a number of towns in and around Bath by members of the department including Chippenham, Malmesbury and Shepton Mallet. Approximately 2000 operations per year are performed in the department at the hospital.

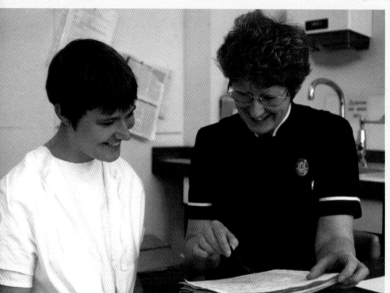

Rebecca Oles came to the RUH to have her wisdom teeth extracted under general anaesthesia as a day case. She was admitted to the unit by Sister Joyce who explained what was going to happen.

An X-ray had already been taken and the last molar (wisdom) teeth (outlined in the picture below) were examined.

Rebecca's teeth were removed under general anaesthesia. The surgery may take up to an hour if the teeth are severely impacted, although some-times it is possible to have your wisdom teeth removed under local anaesthesia alone.

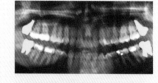

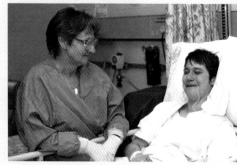

Pain killers were given to Rebecca during her operation and when she recovered from the anaesthetic she had small swabs in place for a few minutes. When these were removed, she was allowed a drink and to go home with her escort/carer. Patients who have had general anaesthesia for day case operations recover quickly. They must still rest at home, however, and avoid operating machinery or equipment (driving a car for instance) for 48 hours to ensure that there are no residual effects from the anaesthetic drugs.

Doctors

The doctors at the RUH account for only 11% of all the people who work at the hospital.

As well as around 120 Consultants on the medical staff, the hospital employs a large number of trainee doctors who will become tomorrow's Consultants.

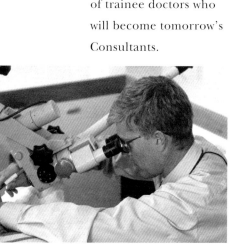

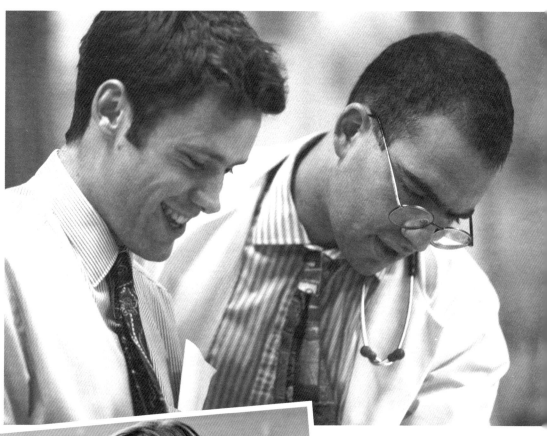

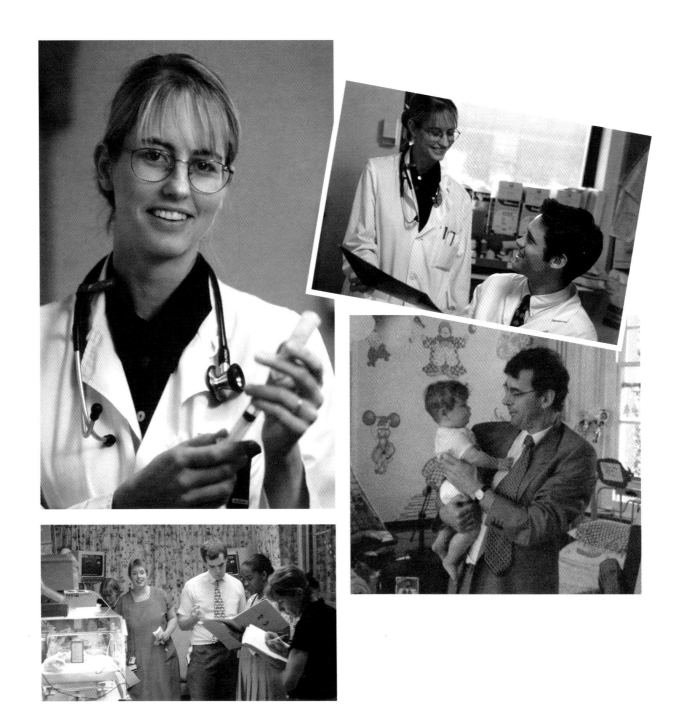

Microbiology

The Department of Microbiology provides a service not only to the RUH but to all our local GPs and Community Hospitals. The laboratory also helps to investigate outbreaks of gastroenteritis (food poisoning) or other infectious diseases in the community such as meningitis. As well as this, the microbiologists support the work of those in public health who might, for instance, be helping to check that restaurants or those that handle food meet acceptable levels of hygiene. When the waters of the Roman spas in Bath are reopened to the public, the Public Health Laboratory Service will work closely with others to ensure that the water remains safe for bathing. The microbiology lab currently processes around 160 000 specimens a year.

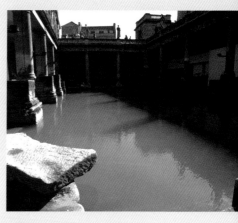

Most of the time in the RUH the microbiologists are to be found on the wards helping other doctors to decide how best to manage patients with infective conditions. Nowhere is this more important than on the Intensive Therapy Unit (ITU) where patients with servere infections are treated.

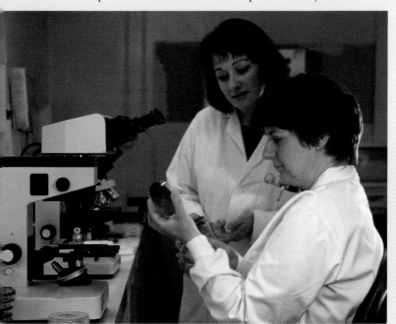

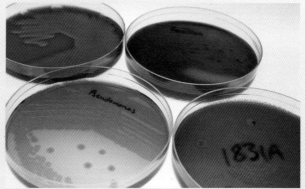

Here Consultant Microbiologist Kim Jacobson (standing) and Clinical Microbiologist Sue Murray discuss the findings from a blood sample taken from a patient on the ITU. They and their colleagues examine blood, swabs, and samples of body secretions for evidence of growth of bacteria and other organisms. The specimens are plated on to agar (nutrient jelly) containing different colour indicators. These colours change in the presence of certain bacteria or other organisms.

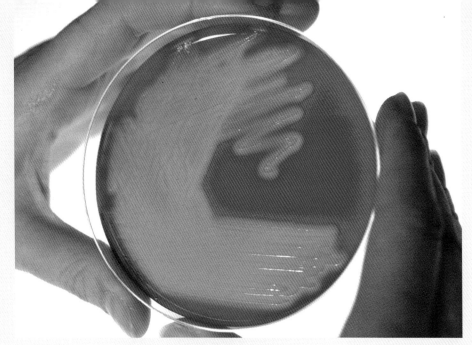

(Left) In this petri dish the bacteria have produced a toxin which has broken down the red blood agar and produced a clear halo around the colonies.

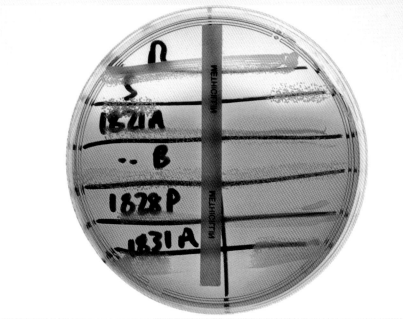

(Above) A colony of bacteria growing in a strip across the top of the dish. It has turned the agar yellow, this helps identify the bacteria as Staphylococcus aureus. Running down the centre of the dish is a strip of paper impregnated with antibiotics. If the organism grows right up to the strip it is resistant to that antibiotic. In this case the S.aureus is resistant to methicillin (so called MRSA, often referred to by the press as the superbug).

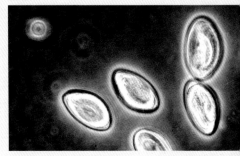

(Above) The ova (eggs) of the parasite Enterobius vermicularis (the threadworm) are seen directly under the phase contrast microscope. This is a very common infection in children and causes itching around the anus especially at night. A strip of sticking tape placed over the child's anus at bedtime will often show the eggs or even the tiny white worm stuck to it when removed in the morning.

Intensive Therapy Unit

The Intensive Therapy Unit (ITU) admits around 500 patients each year. There are no age limits to intensive therapy and each patient is assessed individually on their suitability for admission.

Some of the patients are admitted electively following major surgery with a bed booked for them prior to the operation commencing. Others come to the unit as emergencies after being severely injured in road traffic accidents. The ITU also admits patients with pneumonia or suffering from over-whelming infection.

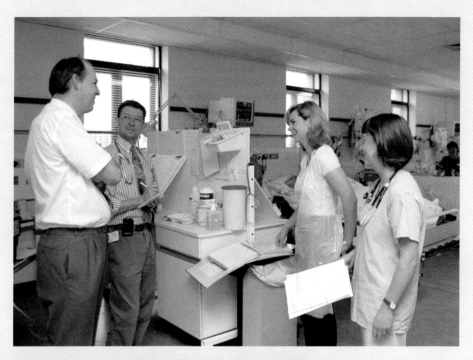

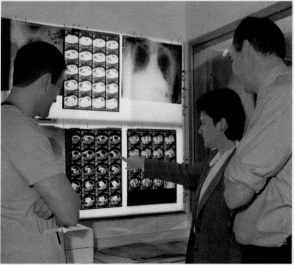

The patient's care is managed and coordinated by the group of six ITU Consultants but specialists from all areas of the hospital are involved as and when required.

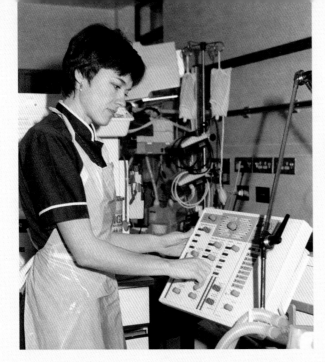

(Above) Sophisticated monitoring systems are essential to ensure that all life supporting functions such as respiration, heart rate, blood pressure, kidney and liver function are optimised for each patient. Equipment used to do this is inevitably very expensive. For example, each ITU bed space must be equipped with a machine to take over the patients respiration (a ventilator) and each ventilator costs around £36 000.

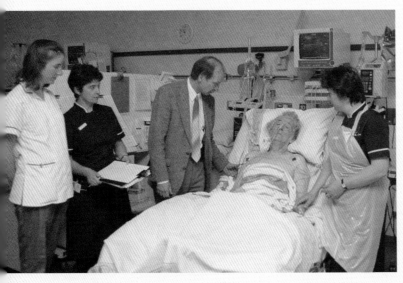

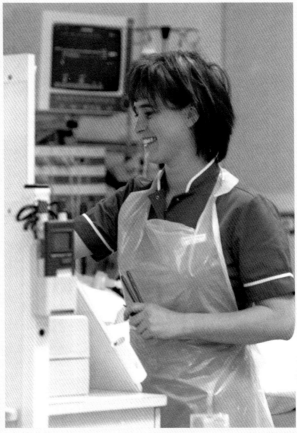

(Above) ITU can be a frightening environment for both patients and relatives. The staff of the unit strive to provide a wholistic approach to patient care, attending not only to the medical needs of the critically ill but also the psychological and spiritual aspects of being a patient or relative on ITU.

(Left) The day to day care of each patient also involves physio-therapists, dieticians and other professional groups in order to provide the very best opportunity for recovery from critical illness. Here the acute pain team are adjusting a patient's pain relief.

Outpatient Investigation

Of course not everyone at the RUH is admitted as an inpatient. Far from it in fact. Many more patients are seen and undergo tests and investigations each year as outpatients. Even those scheduled to have operations are investigated and prepared for their surgery on an outpatient basis. Doctors from the RUH undertake outpatient clinics in the community hospitals around Bath and in some of the General Practitioner's surgeries.

Here are three pictures of patients having tests as outpatients.

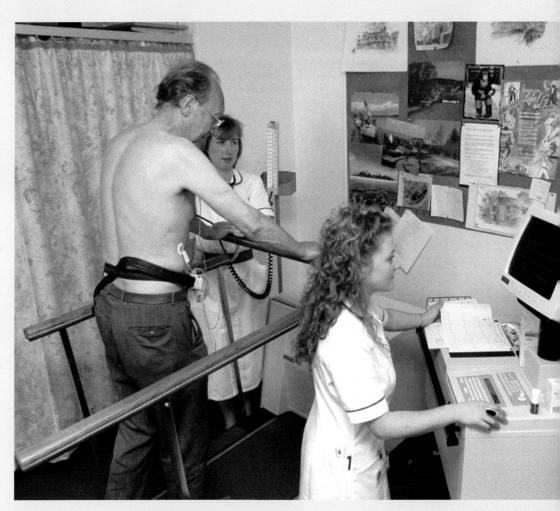

Mr Frederick Chapman is undergoing an exercise ECG as part of the tests performed to try and find out why he was suffering chest pain. Mr Chapman had to exercise on a treadmill whilst a recording of the electrical activity of his heart was taken. This recording was then examined for any evidence of heart disease.

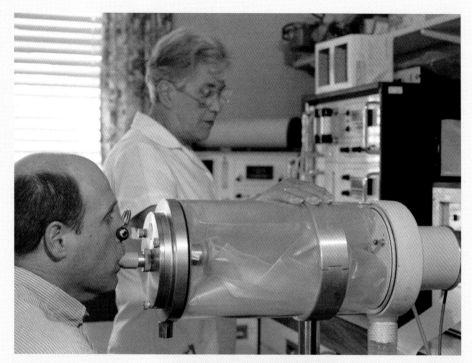

Mr Michael Bees was becoming increasingly short of breath when he exerted himself despite being a keen sportsman. The medical team at the RUH who were asked to see him asked him to attend the Pulmonary Physiology Lab where he underwent lung function tests. These tests showed that Mr Bees' lung capacity was much reduced and helped guide his treatment. After a course of medication, Mr Bees' breathing is now considerably improved.

Mr Harold Skull, who lives in Chippenham, suffered a heart attack in the Autumn of 1996. As part of the investigation of how well his heart had recovered an echocardiogram was performed some months later. During this test a probe is used to bounce soundwaves off the structures of Mr Skull's heart. It is quite painless but allows a picture of the heart as it beats and moves to be recorded. Using a computer, the machine is also able to calculate flow of blood through the heart and even pressure across the heart's valves.

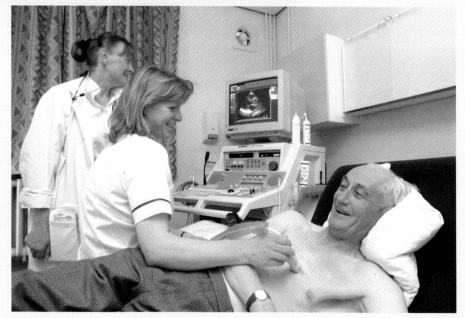

A Lifetime of Learning

Throughout their professional life everyone in the health service continues to learn and develop. Education thus plays a major part in the work of the RUH.

Medical students from University Medical schools in Bristol, Southampton, Oxford and other cities spend time on clinical attachments in Bath.

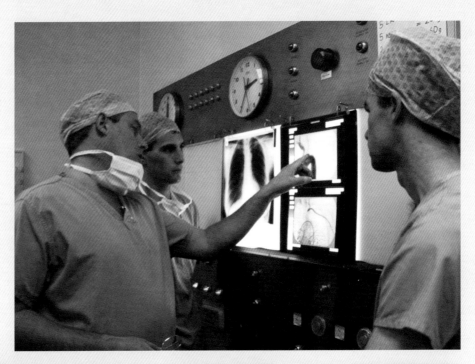

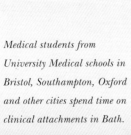

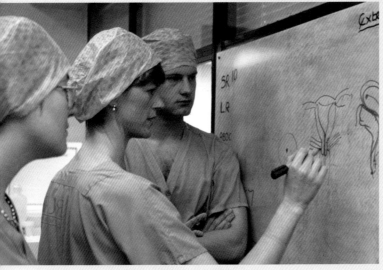

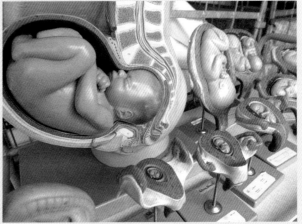

The workload at the RUH is large and provides excellent learning opportunities for students studying to become tomorrow's doctors.

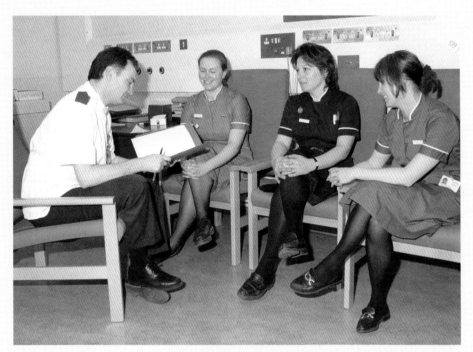

As well as medical students the hospital offers practical experience for a wide variety of health care professionals in training including nurses, physiotherapists, midwives, and health service managers. Continuing education for staff already qualified and working at the RUH is equally important. This may take the form of informal tutorials, case studies, audit meetings, or more formal conferences or courses.

Patients too need to be informed about their condition, what their diagnosis means, how best to cope with it and what treatment may be appropriate.

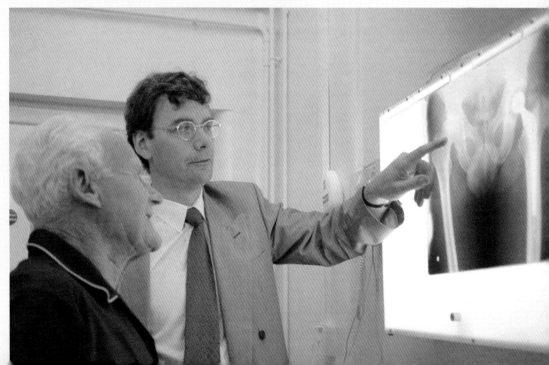

Nurses

The largest group of employees at the RUH are the nursing staff. Approximately 40% of the entire workforce are employed as nurses.

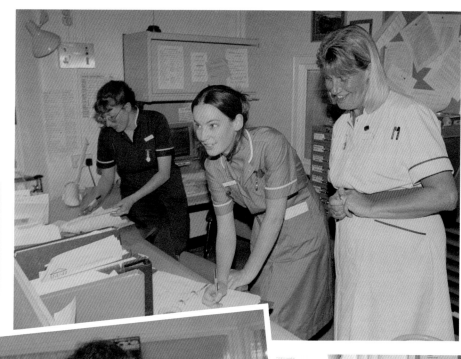

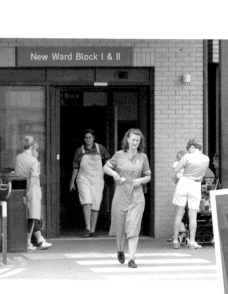

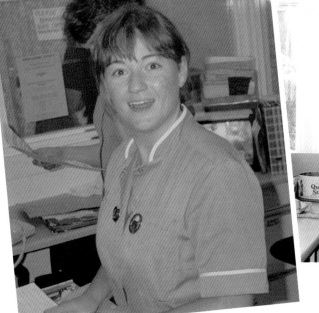

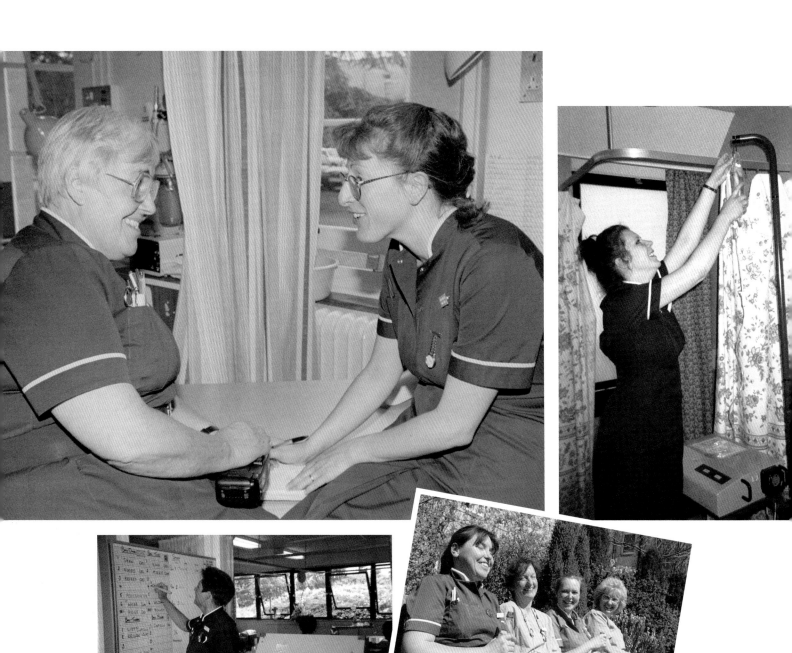

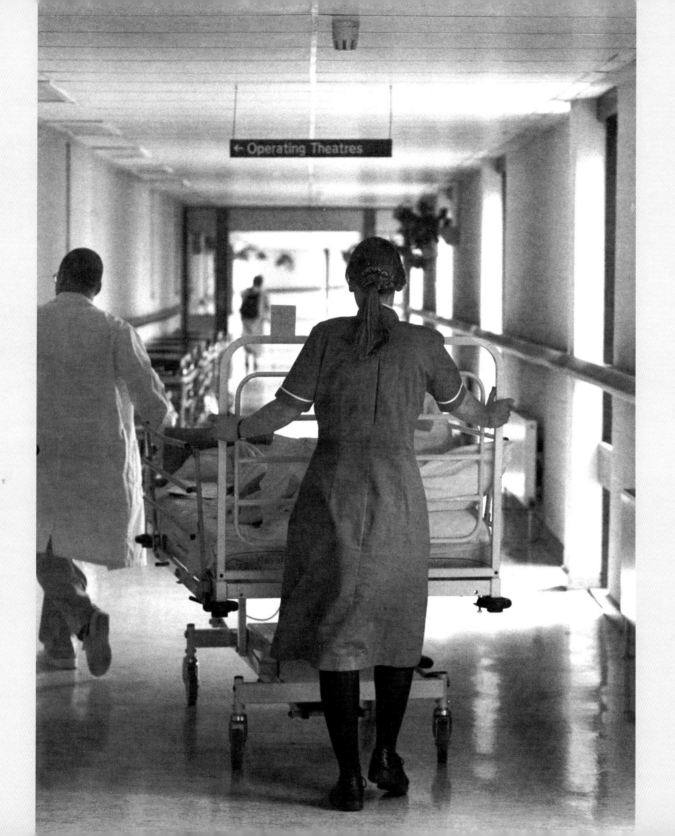

Operating Theatres

There are 14 operating theatres at the RUH in which all types of surgery, with the exception of cardio-thoracic, neurological, and complex paediatric operations, are undertaken. There are two theatres dedicated to day surgery and patients go home after a suitable recovery period on the same day as their operation. Surgeons at the RUH continue to under-take more and more surgery on a day case basis and when the site redevelopment is complete there will be four day surgery theatres in a brand new day surgery unit. The main inpatient theatre suite houses eight theatres, with two theatres dedicated to emergency operations 24 hours a day. Around 23 000 operations a year are undertaken at the RUH.

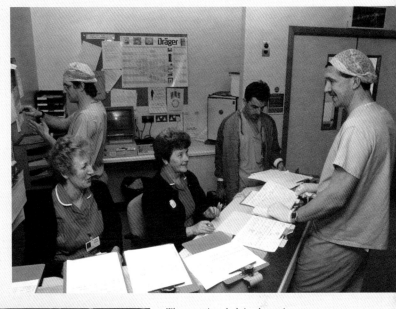

The reception desk in the main theatre suite is the nerve centre for these theatres. Patients are sent for from the wards when it is approaching the time for their operation and checked in to the department to ensure that the correct patient for each theatre has arrived.

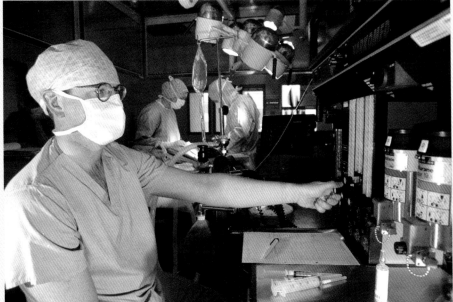

Consultant Anaesthetist Dr Alex Mayor makes fine adjustments to a patient's anaesthetic during the course of their operation.

41

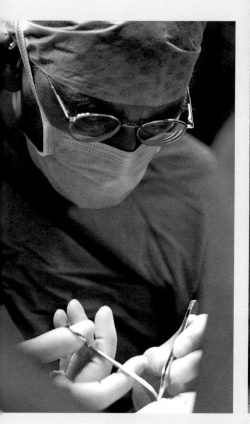

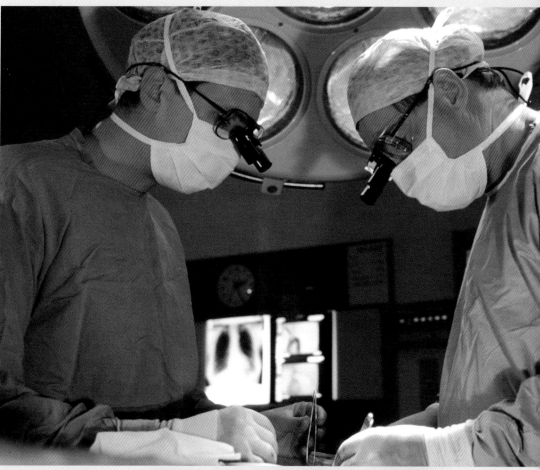

(Above left) Mr Cled Jones, Consultant Orthopaedic Surgeon, using delicate instruments to repair a severed tendon in a wrist.

(Above right) Surgical operations require teams of doctors, nurses, and other healthcare professionals to work together closely. Here Professor Michael Horrocks and one of the surgical trainees operate on a patient's blocked artery.

(Right) Consultant Surgeon Mr Robin Smith operating to remove a patient's gall bladder using so-called key-hole techniques (laparoscopic cholecystectomy).

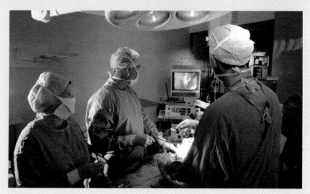

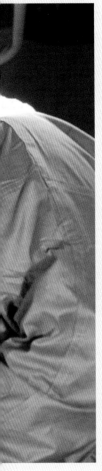

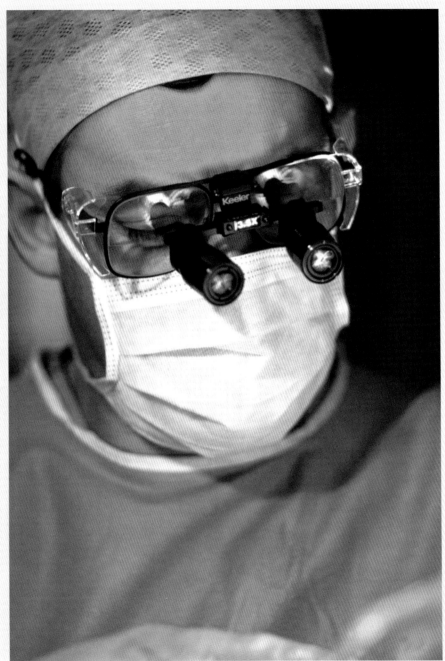

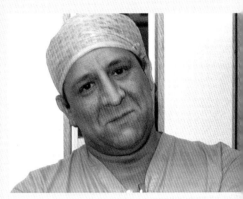

(Above) Senior ODA
(Operating Department
Assistant) John Hughes.

(Left) Vascular Surgeon
Professor Michael Horrocks.

43

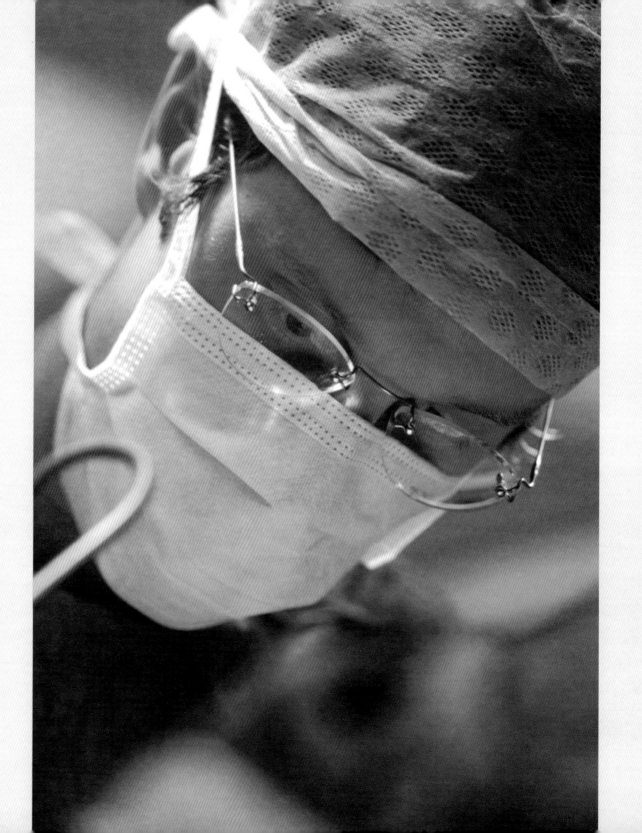

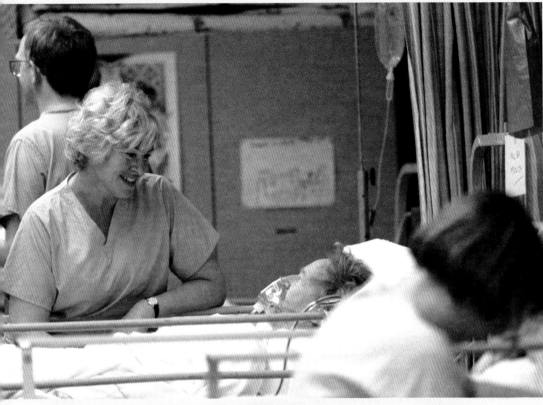

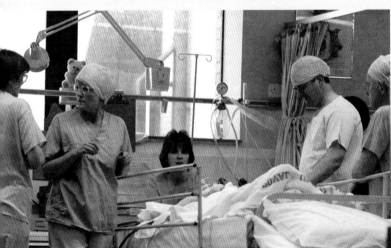

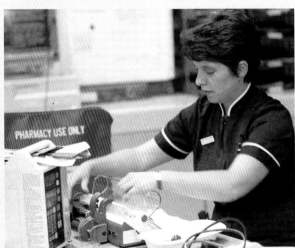

(Left) Recovery Sister Maggie Hill checks that her patient is comfortable and that the vital signs are stable.

(Below left) Following completion of their operation patients are cared for in the recovery room.

(Below right) Sister Brenda Simmons heads the acute pain team which helps inpatients, including those who have had operations, to control their pain.

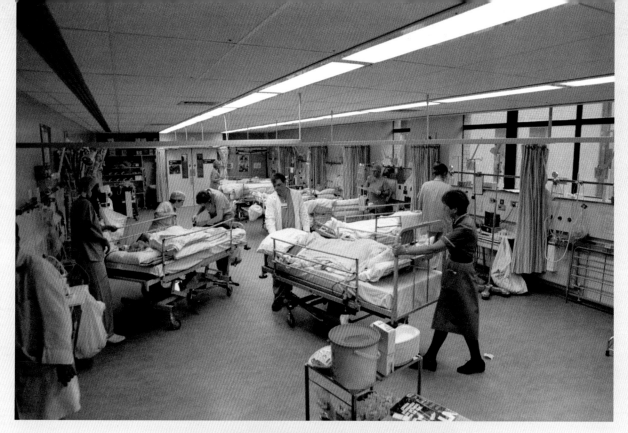

(Above) When patients are fully awake and free from pain they are collected from recovery by their ward nurse.

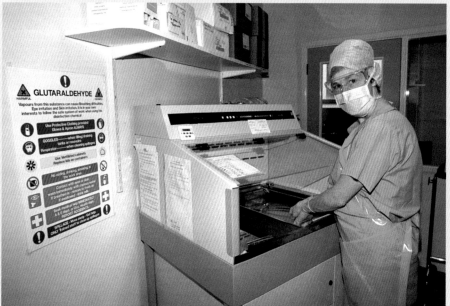

(Left) All instruments used during operations that are not disposable are thoroughly cleaned and sterilised before being used again.

(Right) Medical gases for use in the operating theatres.

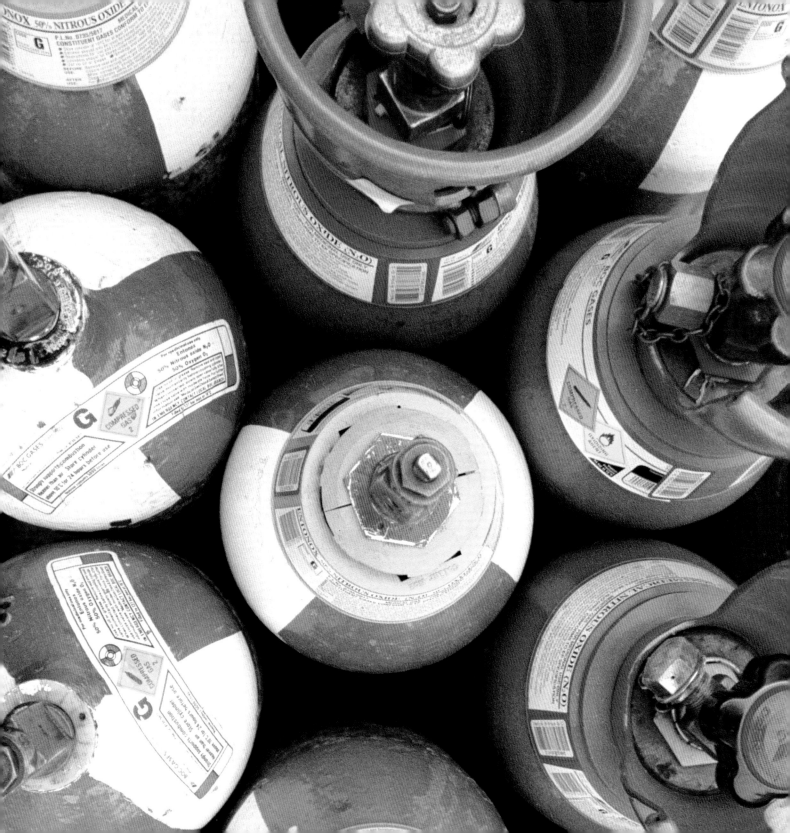

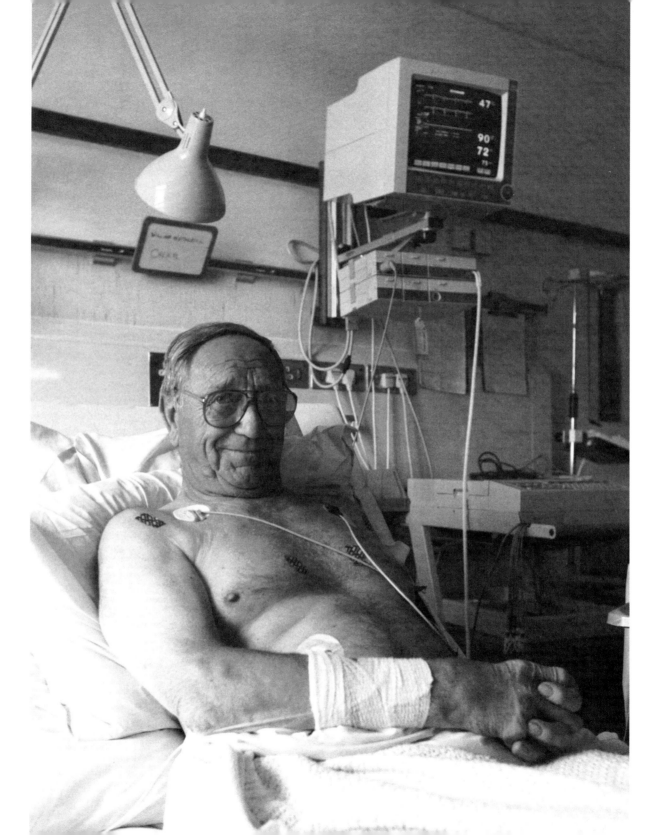

The Patients

The patients that the RUH serves live not only in Bath but in the towns and villages that lie around the city. Some of our patients may live as far away as 25 miles. People treated at the hospital tend to be either children or aged over 65, the latter accounting for 36% of our patients.

In order that the RUH continues to offer the kind of healthcare that our local population require, a doctor in Public Health Medicine has been appointed to work at the hospital. Dr Alison Graham is one of the first Consultants in the country in Public Health Medicine to be appointed to a post in an acute hospital. Alison works closely with our General Practitioners and Health Authorities to ensure that the hospital remains responsive to the health needs of our patients. Many of our patients joined in with our photographic day and some of them are pictured here.

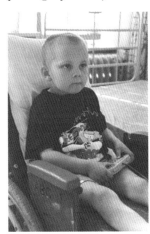

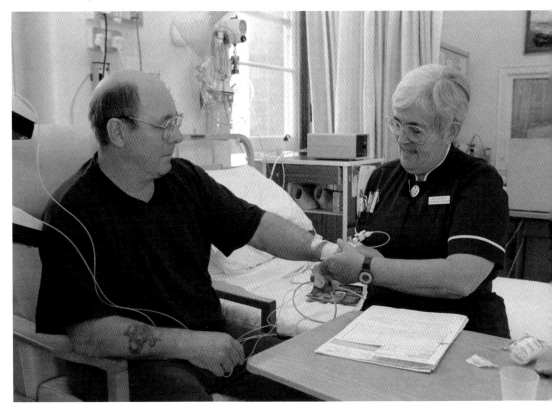

The RUH treats around 50 000 inpatients and
173 000 outpatients per year. Patients may be in
hospital for as little as a day, or, more unusually,
for many weeks.

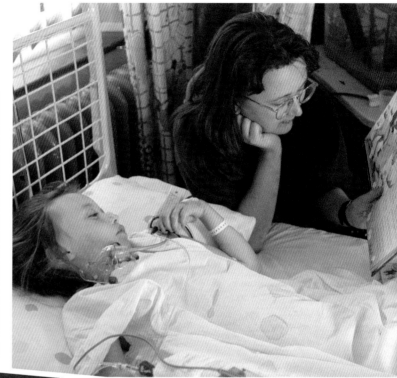

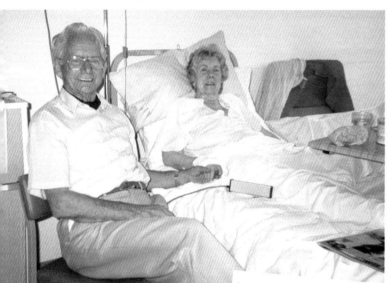

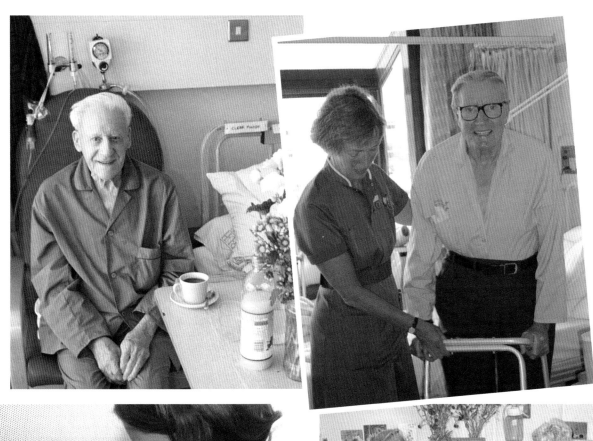

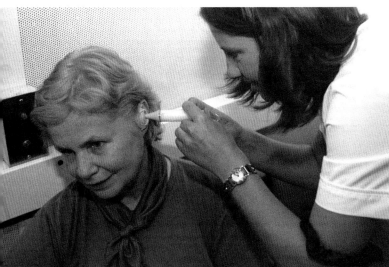

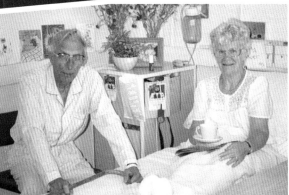

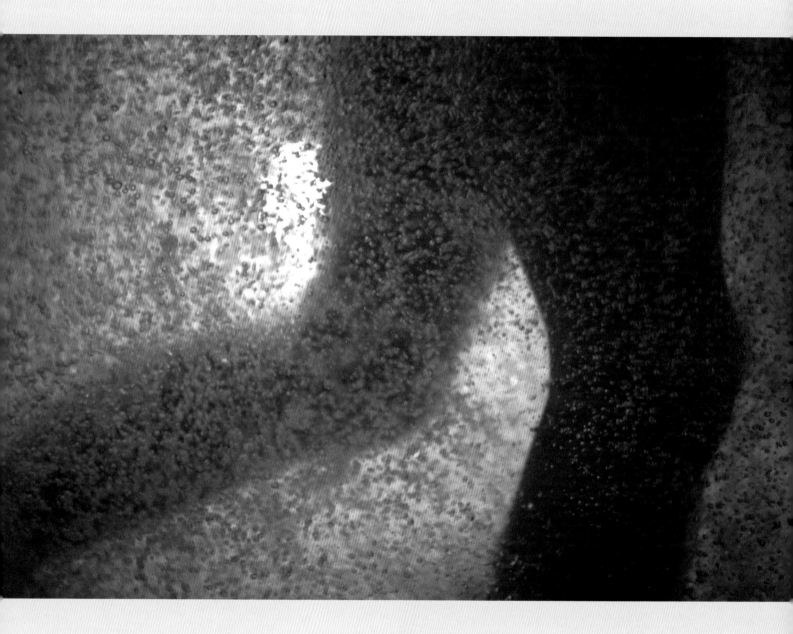

Physiotherapy

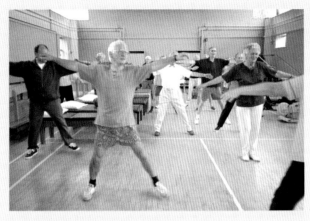

Around 10 000 patients are treated by the hospital's physiotherapists each year. Approximately 7000 of these are inpatients whilst the remaining 3000 are treated on an outpatient basis. Physiotherapy is essential in the recovery of patients with a wide range of medical and surgical conditions.

A number of different treatment techniques are used but one of the most unusual is the Aquaciser. This is an underwater treadmill which allows the patient to undertake quite hard physical exercise without fully weight-bearing. The patient enters the tank and the sealed door is closed behind them. Warm water is then pumped into the tank and the treadmill started. Exercise in this way is particularly helpful for patients who are recovering from leg fractures or older patients with painful joints who may find exercise difficult or impossible. Superintendent Physiotherapist Jim Grant is supervising Benjamin Edwards in the Aquaciser. Ben fractured both bones in his lower leg whilst

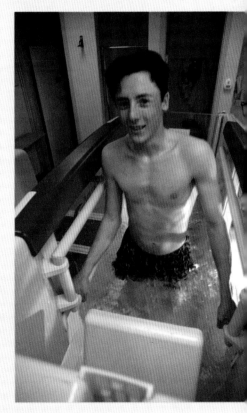

mountain biking on a hill near Devizes. He was airlifted by the air ambulance from the scene of his accident and admitted to the hospital. Ben is a keen sportsman and wanted to regain his full physical fitness as part of his recovery.

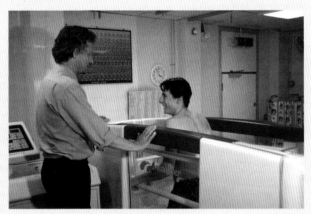

Pharmacy

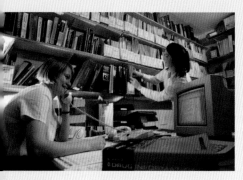

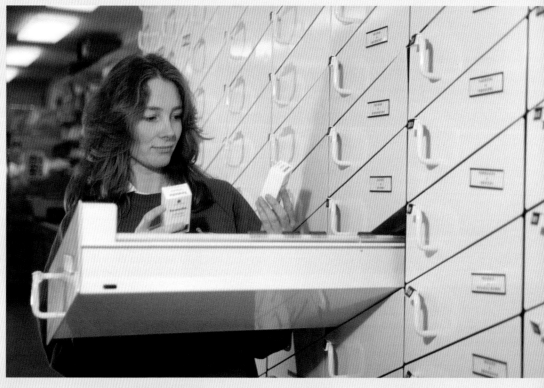

A drug information service is provided by the Pharmacy at the RUH, not only for doctors and nurses who work at the hospital but it is also freely accessible to General Practitioners and by chemists in the Bath area.

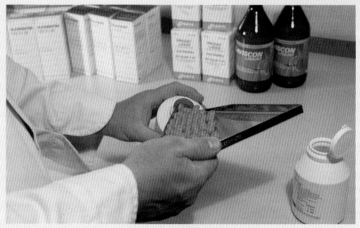

Drugs are stored in a variety of drawer and cupboard systems prior to being dispensed. They are then placed in red delivery bags which are sealed for delivery to the wards and other clinical areas in the hospital. The Pharmacy at the RUH dispenses over 20 000 items per month.

Staff at the Pharmacy maintain a stock level of regularly used preparations with regular deliveries to clinical areas.

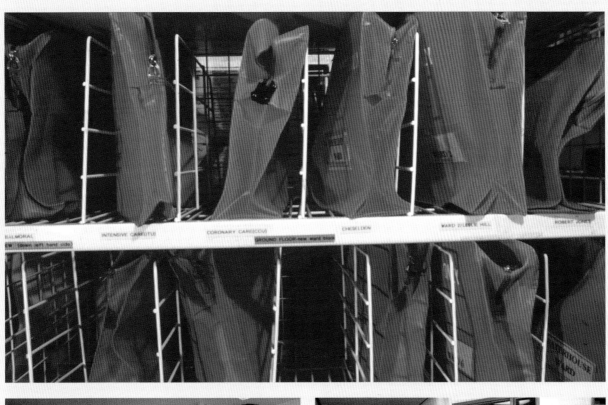

BALMORAL   INTENSIVE CARE(ITU)   CORONARY CARE(CCU)   CHESELDEN   WARD 2/LESLIE HILL   ROBERT JONES

EW (down left hand side)   GROUND FLOOR-new ward block

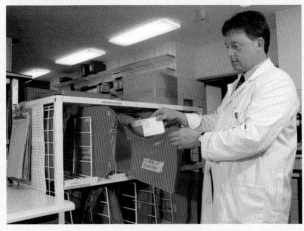

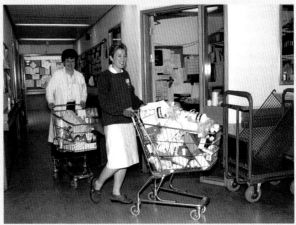

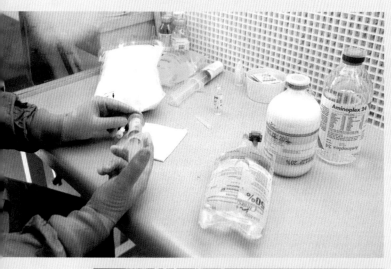

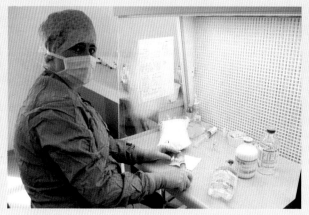

The Pharmacy is responsible for making up feeding solutions and anti-cancer chemotherapy drugs which are then administered directly into patient's veins. These solutions must be prepared under strict sterile conditions. All additions to the basic solutions must therefore be made in the Pharmacy before being sent to the ward.

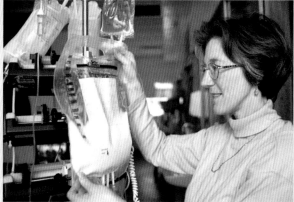

(Above) These three pictures show a bag of intravenous feeding solution being prepared and checked. It contains all the nutrition that an adult requires in 24 hours.

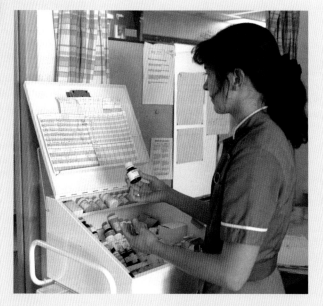

The Pharmacy at the RUH also dispenses and delivers drugs for administration to both inpatients and outpatients to family planning clinics, dental practices, St Martin's Hospital and the Royal National Hospital for Rheumatic Diseases in Bath.

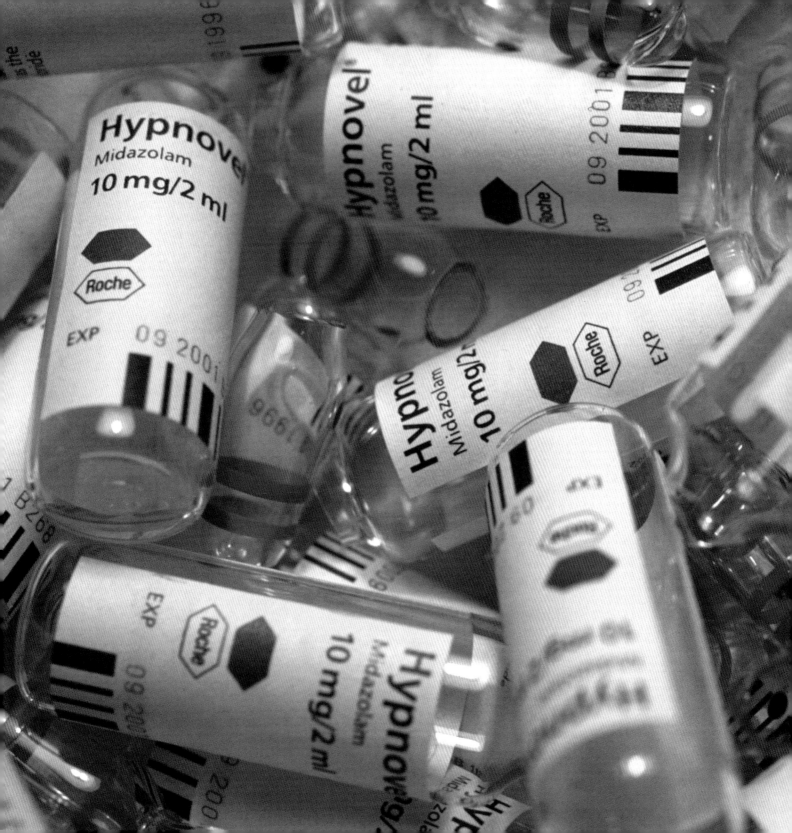

Unsung heroes

The non-medical support staff play a vital part in the running of the hospital, without them the RUH simply could not function. They perform a variety of roles, just a few of which are featured here.

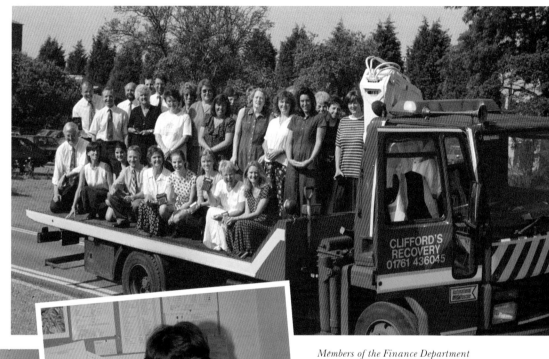

Members of the Finance Department

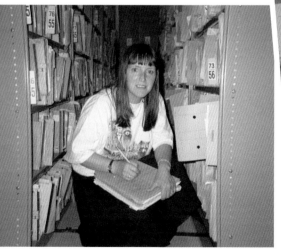

Shirley Cooper, Medical Records Assistant

Pauline Francis, Senior Pathology Receptionist

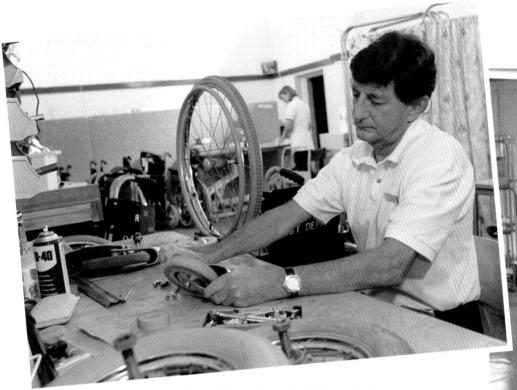

Richard Heath, Occupational Therapy Assistant

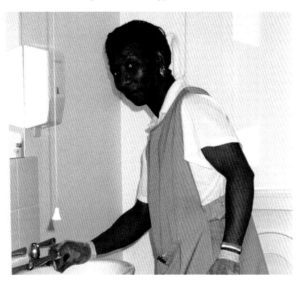

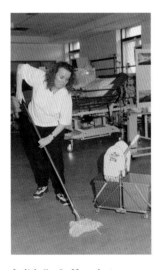

Judith Craft, Housekeeper

George Hale, Stores Coordinator

Elaine Thomas, Housekeeper

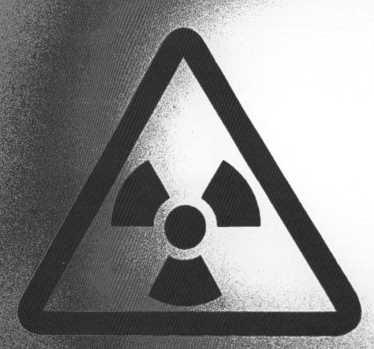

Radiology

The Department of Radiology at the RUH produces all manner of images to assist in the diagnosis and treatment of both inpatients and outpatients. The department also supports colleagues in general practice with their own imaging needs. Indeed, GPs and patients have welcomed the pioneering teleradiology between the RUH and Chippenham Community Hospital. This enables a GP in the Casualty Department at Chippenham to transmit an X-ray image of a suspected fracture, for instance, to the RUH for an immediate expert opinion.

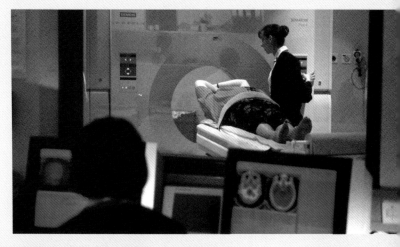

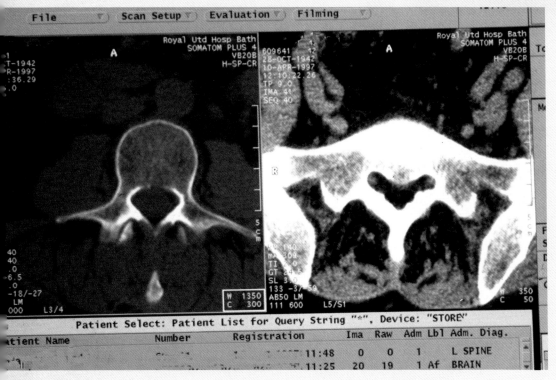

Here a patient is undergoing a CT scan of her back for investigation of back pain. The resulting scans show a section through the bony part of the patient's back.

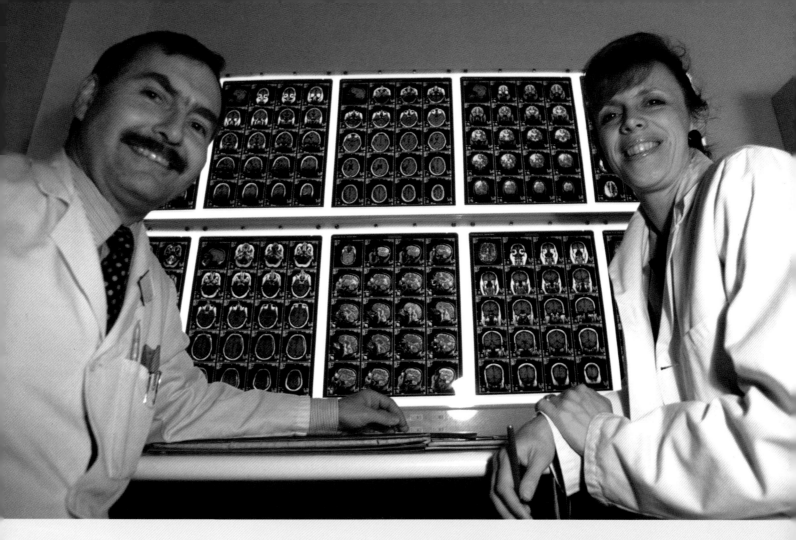

Consultant Radiologists
Drs Louise Robinson and
Mike Noakes provide expert
opinions of the scans that have
been taken earlier in the day.

The RUH boasts state-of-the-art CT and MRI scanners. Computerised tomography (CT) is an imaging technique using X-rays which allows sections of the body to be viewed as though they were slices of bread from a loaf. If the slices are put together one after the other then the body can be viewed as a whole. The images are more detailed than with plain X-ray and approximately 100 patients per week are booked in for a CT scan. As well as this, the scanner is being used increasingly to obtain rapid diagnostic information in emergency patients.

MRI stands for magnetic resonance imaging and does not use X-rays at all. This is an imaging technique which utilises a magnet which is 10 000 times stronger than the earth's magnetic field. Because the magnet is so strong it is important that certain metal objects are kept well away from the magnetic field. This means that it is not a technique suitable for patients who have had, for example, cardiac pacemakers implanted, metallic clips placed across arteries which have bled inside the brain, or have metallic foreign bodies in them following accidents at work. Patients and staff are also reminded to leave their credit cards outside the field as the magnet will wipe all the electronic data stored on them!

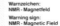

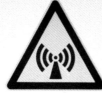
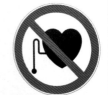

MAGNETOM

Warnzeichen:
NMR - Magnetfeld

Signal attention:
Champ Magnetique RMN

Warning sign:
NMR - Magnetic Field

Símbolo de advertencia:
NMR Champo Magnetico

Warnzeichen:
Hochfrequenzfeld

Signal attention:
Champ Haute Frequence

Warning sign:
High' Frequency Field

Símbolo de advertencia:
Campo de alta Frequencia

Verbotszeichen:
elektromagnetisch beeinflussbare Implantate, z.B. Herzschrittmacher, Defibrillatoren, Hörgeräte, Insulinpumpen, Medikamentendosiergeräte

Danger Symbols:
Danger of Electromagnetic Disturbances Implantations, e.g. Cardiac Pacemaker, Defibrillators, Hearing Instruments, Insulin Pumps, Dosage Devices for Medication

Panneaux d'avertissement:
éléments implantés sensibles aux interférences électromagnétiques, par ex. stimulateurs cardiaques, défibrillateurs, aides auditives, pompes à insuline, doseurs de médicaments

Símbolos de prohibición:
Implantes sensibles a los campos electromagnéticos, p.ej. marcapasos, desfibriladores, audífonos, bombas de insulina, dosificadores de medicamentos

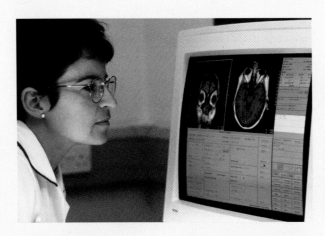

(Above left) Whilst CT scans are good for showing up bony problems, magnetic resonance images are especially helpful for diagnosing soft tissue abnormalities. This means it is frequently used to image the brain and spinal cord and here Superintendent Radiographer Di Pressdee is planning a brain scan.

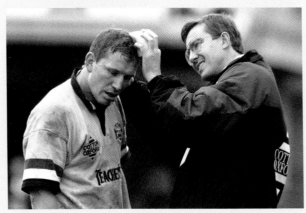

(Left) Because of its benefits in soft tissue diagnosis, MRI is also often employed when investigating sports injuries and it is not uncommon to find a member of the Bath Rugby squad booked in for an urgent scan!

Radioisotope scanning is another imaging technique available at the RUH. Most organs in the body, as well as bone, can be imaged in this way and two gamma cameras including a new dual-headed model are used to produce around 4000 scans a year.

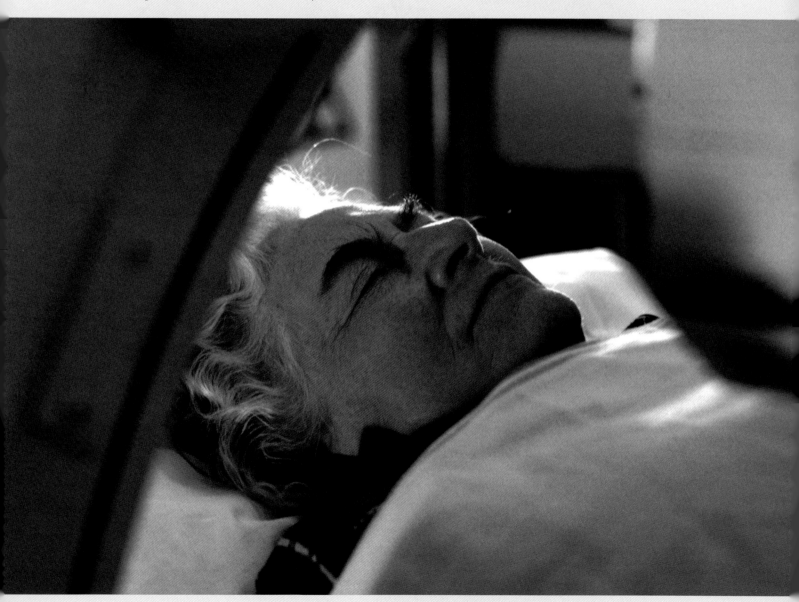

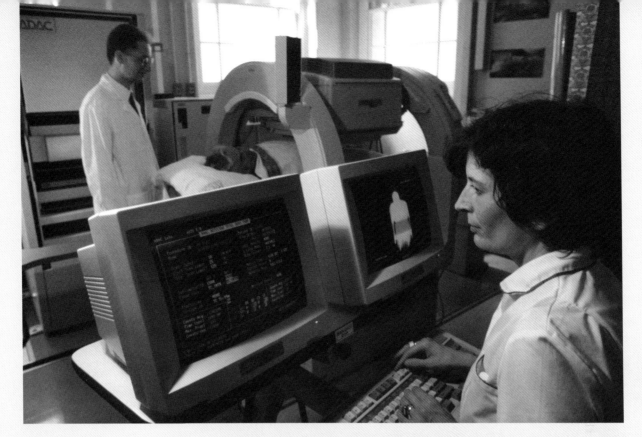

(Above) Chief Radioisotope Technician Kathy Bunnett is ensuring that the patient is correctly positioned in the dual-head scanner.

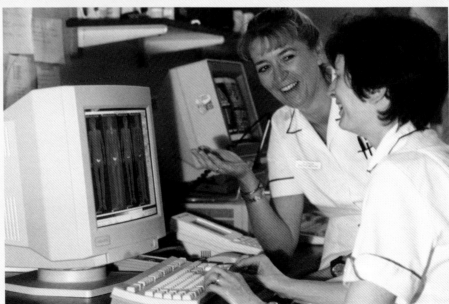

(Right) Kathy and her colleague Jo Phillips plan a bone scan.

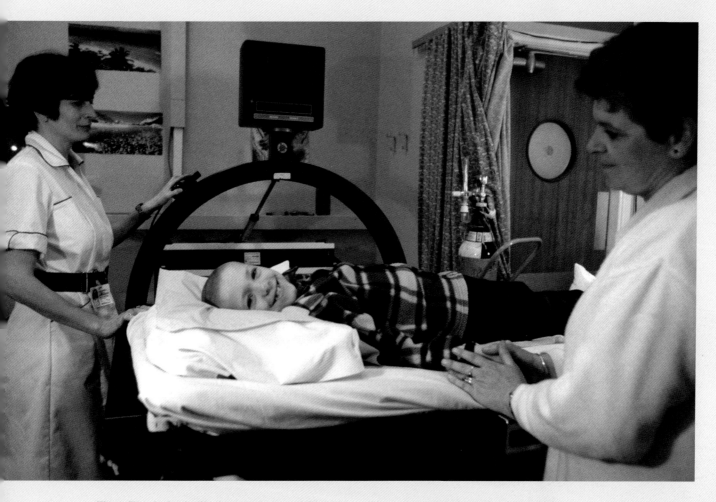

This is Timothy Bowler-Witt having a bone scan. Timmy was well known around the hospital as he was a frequent visitor. He was found to be suffering from lymphoblastic leukaemia and underwent courses of treatment using chemotherapy and radiotherapy as well as bone marrow transplantation. Despite all this and a very aggressive disease Timmy was always a happy and smiling 9 year old whenever he came to the RUH. Sadly, Timmy's disease could not be controlled and he died in the summer of 1997.

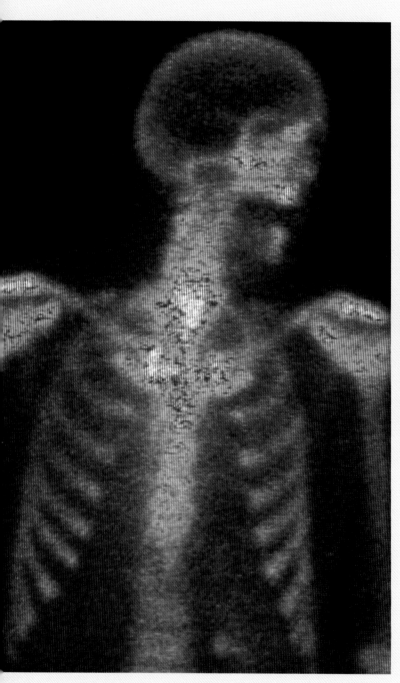

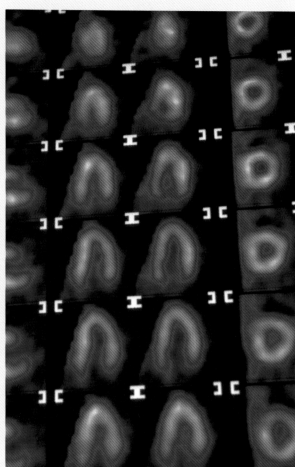

(Above) This series of scans have been taken to look at the blood supply to the main chamber in the heart.

(Left) This is a bone scan which we have enhanced to produce a rather unusual image of the upper body.

Allied Professions

There are many professions allied to the medical and scientific staff at the RUH. Here are just a few of them.

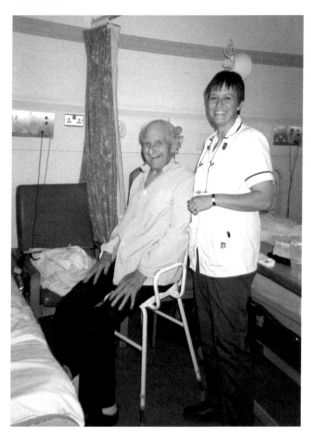

Anne Hastings, Senior Occupational Therapist.

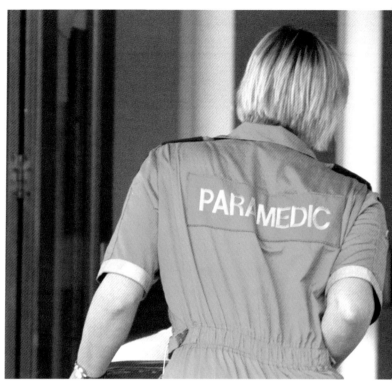

Louise, one of the Avon Ambulance Paramedics.

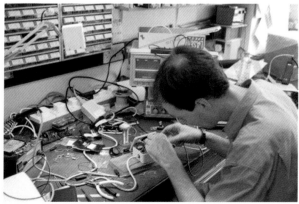

Peter Dicken, Electronics Engineer in Medical Physics.

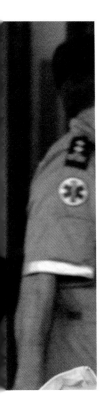

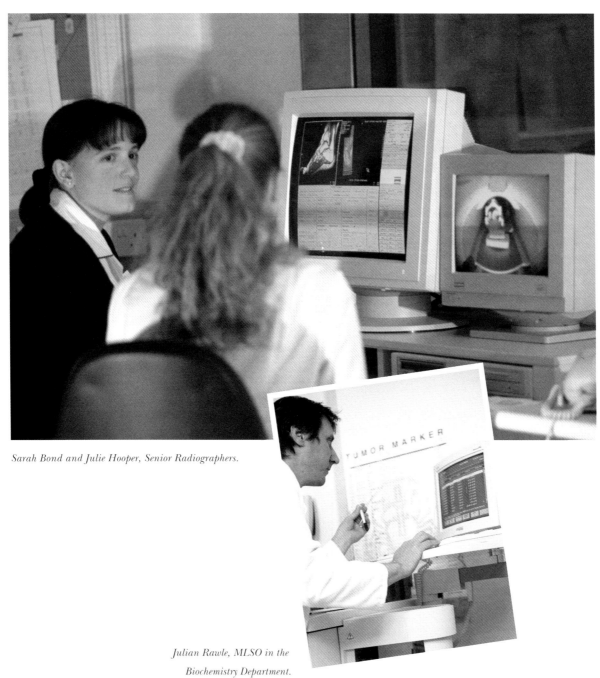

Sarah Bond and Julie Hooper, Senior Radiographers.

Julian Rawle, MLSO in the
Biochemistry Department.

Local support

The RUH is fortunate in receiving the support of a large network of voluntary groups, volunteers and friends from the local community such as the League of Friends, the Women's Royal Voluntary

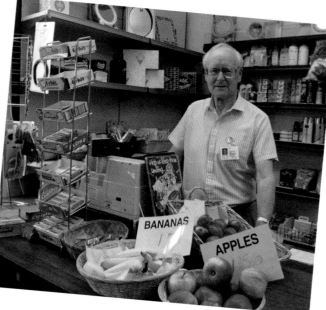

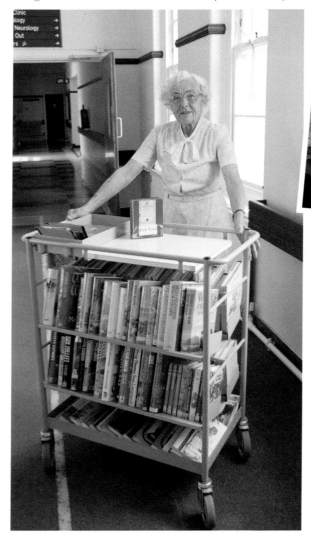

Service, the Bath Cancer Unit Support Group, and Bath Hospital Radio. Their contribution to the hospital is invaluable and almost every department and ward within the hospital has at some stage benefited from their generosity. Such groups provide guides at some of the entrances to the hospital, work as volunteers on wards, and raise funds through the hospital shop, conservatory coffee shop, annual fete, tea parties and donations. For those fans of Bath Rugby who are unfortunate enough to miss a home game through being hospitalised in the RUH, Bath Hospital Radio even provide live commentary on Saturday afternoons!

Maternity

Around 5000 babies are born each year in the catchment area of the RUH. The hospital offers obstetric services to the higher risk pregnancies as well as acting as the community hospital for the Bath city deliveries. Approximately 3700 deliveries take place each year at the RUH with the remainder occurring in the seven community units in towns around Bath.

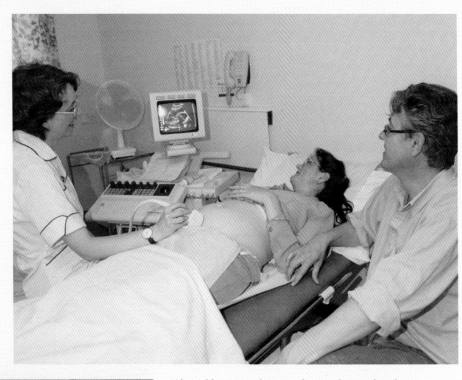

(Above) Most women have an ultrasound scan when they are approximately 20 weeks pregnant. The scan is done at this time as it may show a wide range of abnormalities in the baby should they be present. Here just such a scan is being performed and both parents are able to see the image of their baby on the screen.

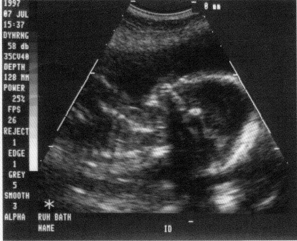

(Left) The scan shows the baby to be lying across the picture with his or her head to the right and the chest with one arm above it reaching to the left.

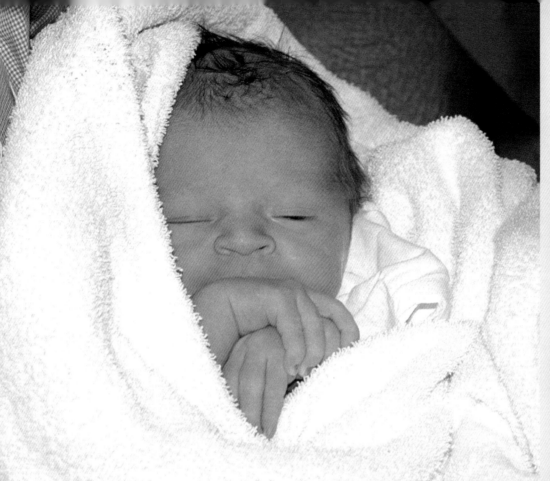

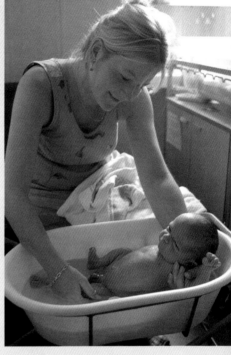

(Above) William Mayor who was born just a few minutes before our photograph. He has been dried off so he doesn't get cold.

A comprehensive maternity service is available at the RUH including physiotherapy specially designed to address the needs of pregnant women. (Right) An antenatal exercise class being undertaken in the warm water of the hydrotherapy pool.

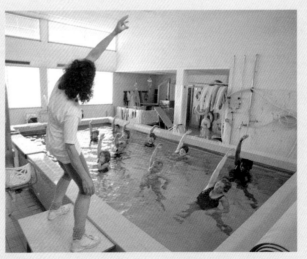

(Above) Parents are encouraged to participate as much as possible in the daily care of their babies whilst they are in hospital so that they may receive advice if they need it on, for instance, how to bathe a newborn baby safely.

(Right) Charlotte Hayde, Mary and Errol's first child, was born at the RUH after 10½ hours of labour.

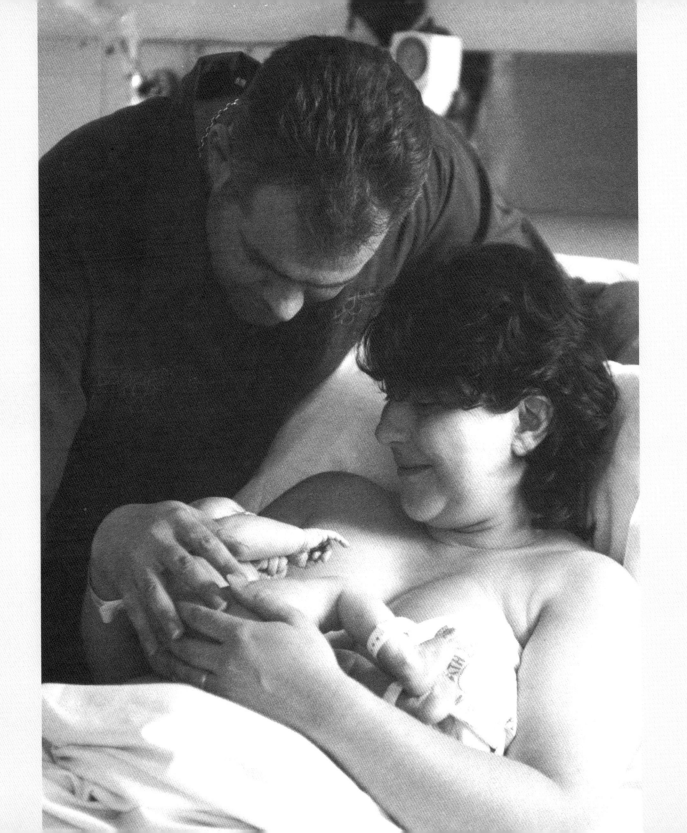

Newborn Intensive Care

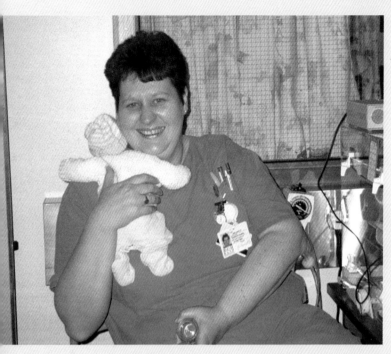

(Above) Nursery Nurse Jan Lovett comforts one of the Unit's patients.

(Right) In this photograph and on the cover of this book Molly Bevan is seen having phototherapy. Molly was born 5 weeks early and her liver did not function adequately shortly after birth. She became jaundiced and the blue light helps eliminate the yellow pigment.

The Newborn Intensive Care Unit (NICU) cares for those newborn babies who require specialist treatment. The unit has 21 cots, four of which are designated for intensive care. Babies admitted to the unit range in age from the minute they were born to one month old or if they were delivered prematurely, one month beyond the date upon which they were expected to have been born. Babies may stay on the unit for just a few hours or for as long as three months for the very premature. NICU is a family centered unit in which parents are encouraged to participate as much as possible. Overnight accommodation is offered to parents in a number of delightfully decorated double and single bedded rooms with kitchen and living facilities immediately adjacent to the unit.

As in the adult Intensive Therapy Unit, the work here goes on day and night, 365 days a year. Care for our youngest patients is provided by teams of doctors and nurses working together. Indeed, the unit pioneered some of the first neonatal nurse practitioners in the country. These are highly trained people whose roles overlap those of nurses and junior doctors. The neonatal nurse practitioners at the RUH are able to insert catheters (tubes) into veins for connection to drip sets, place breathing tubes in the main airway of babies requiring support for their breathing, order blood tests and act on their results, and contribute much to the management of patients on the Unit.

The RUH also operates a neonatal flying squad for the transfer and retrieval of sick babies out of and into the Unit. As with other areas of the hospital, patients may have to travel many miles and the safe transport of sick newborn babies requires specialist knowledge and equipment.

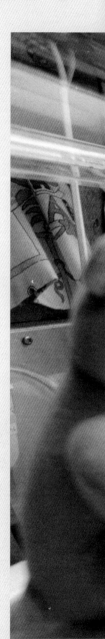

Unit

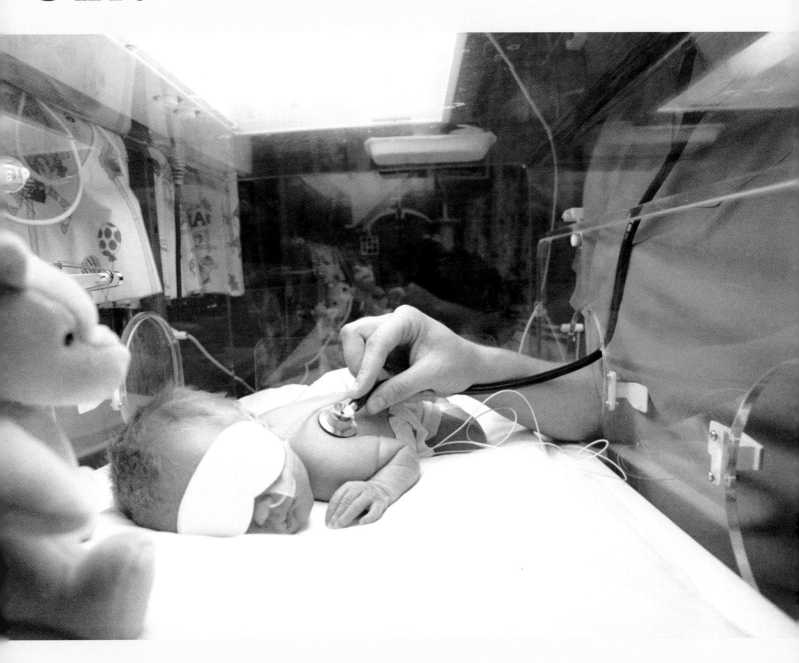

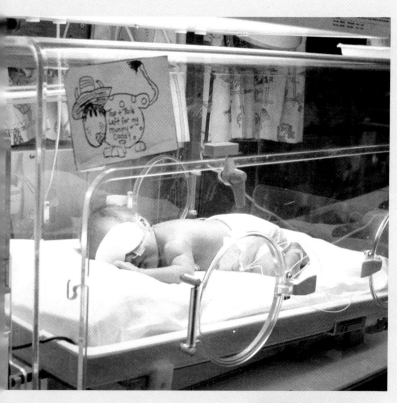

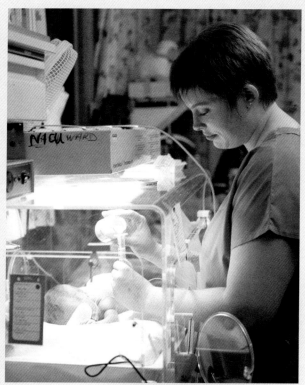

(Clockwise from above)
The notice on the side of the incubator indicates that Molly will be washed and changed (top and tailed) by her mum.

Staff Nurse Catherine Furze attending to Molly.

Molly has a fine feeding tube passed through her nostril to her stomach so that she may be given regular milk feeds.

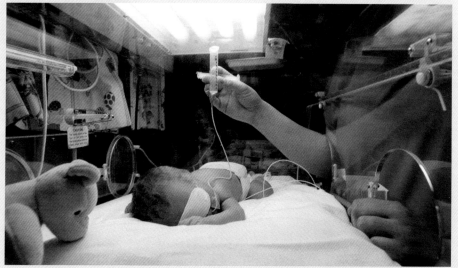

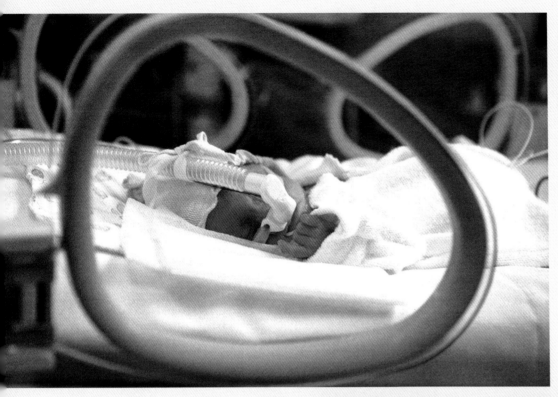

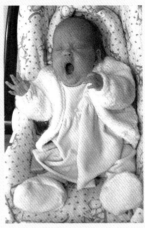

(Above) Rachel stayed on the unit for 86 days during which time she was fed Dawn's expressed milk and has now gone home completely fit and well. She is shown here visiting the hospital some weeks later and has clearly become rather bored with the RUH!

(Above) Rachel Gayfer was born after her mother Dawn had been pregnant for only 25 weeks (a normal pregnancy lasts 40 weeks). She was very premature and weighed only 900 grams (2 lbs) at birth. Rachel's care was thus at the limits of medical expertise.

(Right) Sophie Haynes gets to know her parents whilst receiving help with her breathing from a special type of oxygen delivery system called CPAP.

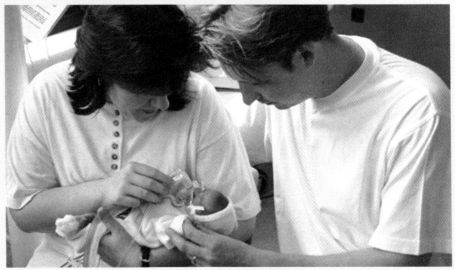

For the children...

When children are admitted to hospital it is essential that we remember to care for the whole child and all his or her needs, not just focus on the cause for their admission. Children at the RUH are cared for by specialist teams who are dedicated to looking after all aspects of the sick child. Parents are encouraged to be part of that team and to be with their children to support them as much as possible. The values and standards of everyone who is associated with the RUH are never more important than when we are looking after sick or injured children.

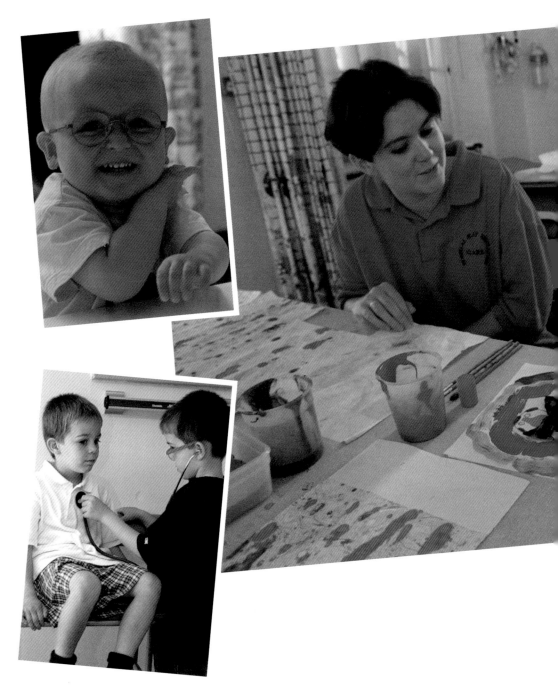

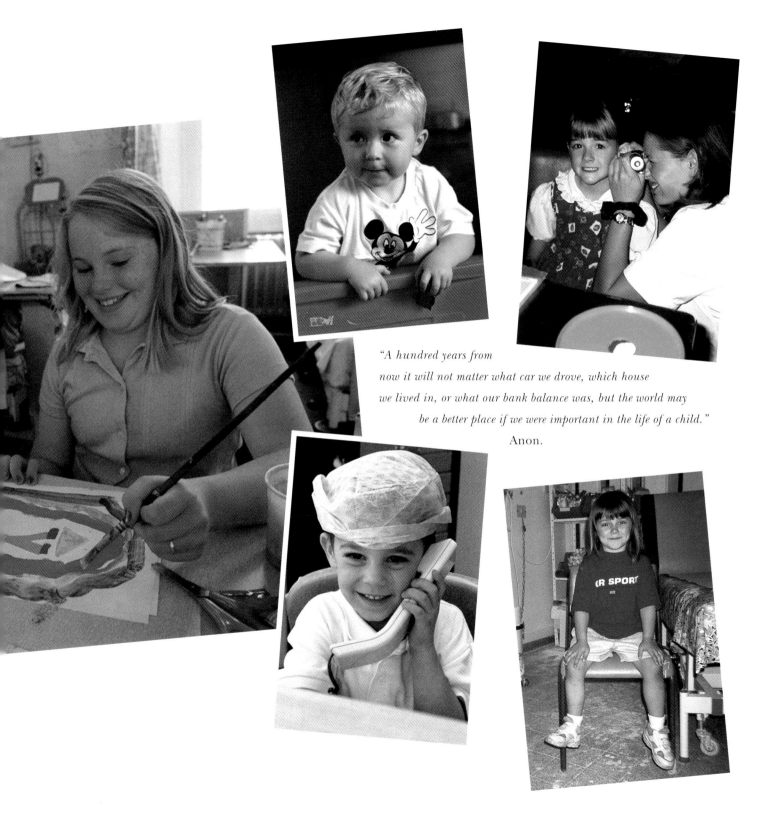

"A hundred years from now it will not matter what car we drove, which house we lived in, or what our bank balance was, but the world may be a better place if we were important in the life of a child."

Anon.

The Eye Unit

The Department of Ophthalmology performs over 2000 procedures per year on patients in the RUH. Patients undergoing eye operations tend to be at the extremes of age. They may be a new born baby or an older patient having, for instance, their cataracts removed. Recently a lady aged 103 years had her cataract removed at the RUH. Approximately 95% of all eye operations are performed under local anaesthesia alone and around 85% of eye operations are undertaken on a day case basis.

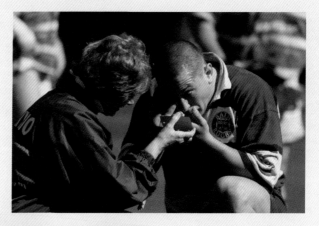

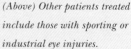

(Above) Other patients treated include those with sporting or industrial eye injuries.

(Left) Consultant Ophthalmological Surgeon Mr Jonathan Griffiths is assessing a patient's eye before discussing treatment options.

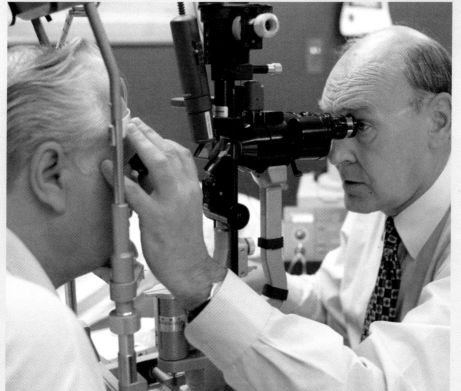

(Right) When eye operations are being performed the eye is viewed through an operating microscope and the image displayed on a TV monitor so that the whole theatre team are aware of the stage of the procedure.

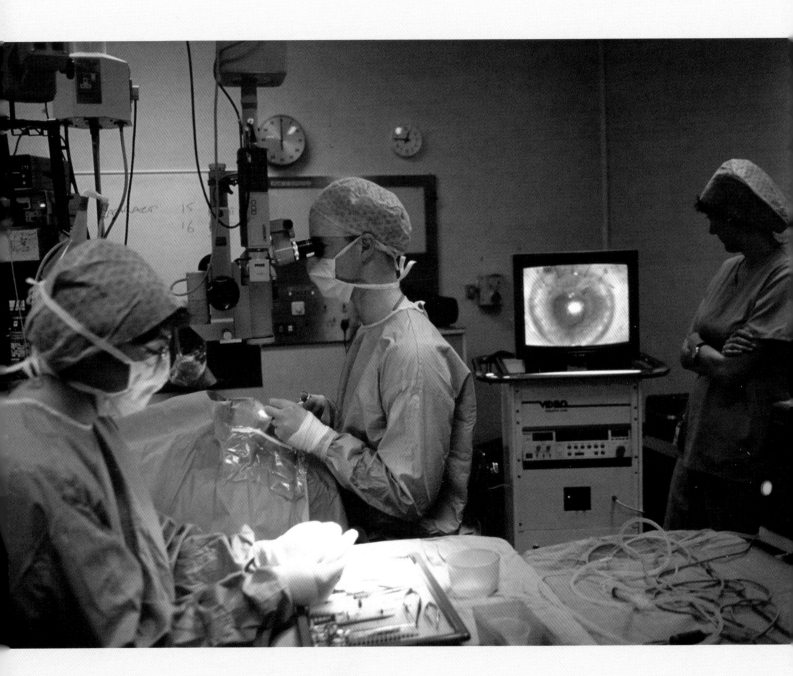

Haematology

Donated blood remains vitally important to many clinical departments in the hospital. A bag of donated blood is used to collect a variety of products, rarely these days is the unit stored and then transfused as whole blood. More usually it is centrifuged (spun at high speed) and the red cells are separated off to be stored. Other products are also collected. These include factors which may help restore normal clotting to patients who are bleeding and antibodies including anti-D antibodies for pregnant women who are Rhesus negative. Donated blood can be stored for up to 42 days. Blood donors can donate blood on site at the RUH as well as at a number of donation centres around Bath.

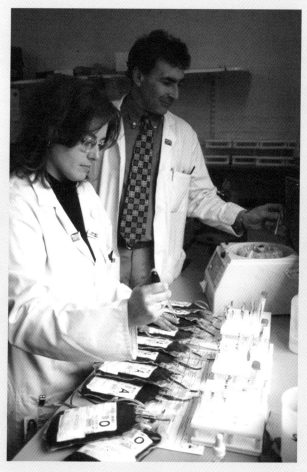

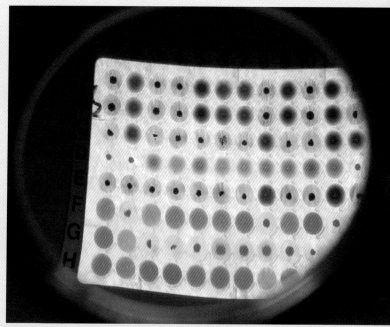

Last year the Department of Haematology cross matched 94 000 units of blood for patients. This involves establishing the blood group of the patient and then testing donated blood against a sample of the patient's blood to ensure compatibility.

(Left) Medical Laboratory Scientific Officers (MLSOs) Richard Gardiner and Amanda Dornan cross matching blood.

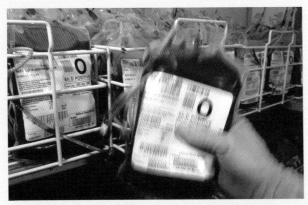

Sometimes blood is required urgently, for instance if a badly injured trauma victim has arrived in A&E or if a patient is losing blood unexpectedly during surgery. Type-specific blood can be ready in 5 minutes to be rushed to the team looking after the patient. A more complete cross match takes 20 minutes to perform.

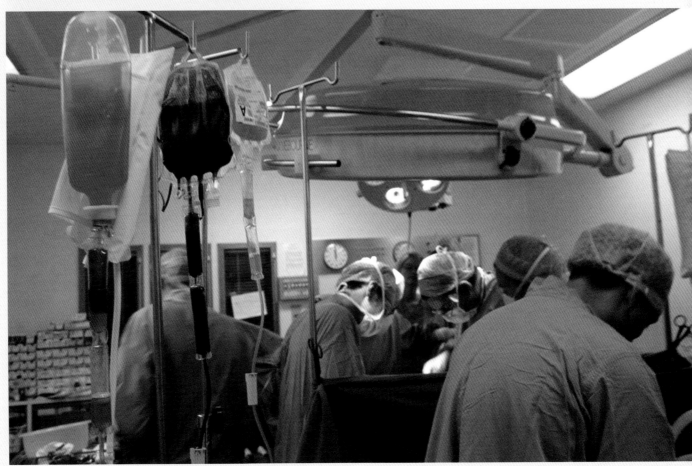

Around 250 units of blood are stored at the hospital at any one time and there are daily deliveries of blood and blood products to the RUH from the Regional Transfusion Service in Bristol.

The Department of Haematology also has two full time Consultant Haematologists who have a busy clinical practice. They help care for patients with a wide range of blood conditions such as anaemia, bleeding disorders and the blood malignancies (e.g. leukaemia and lymphoma). Around 50 new cases of adult blood malignancy are treated at the RUH each year. Treatment for these patients may include outpatient chemotherapy, high dose chemoradiotherapy, or stem cell transplantation.

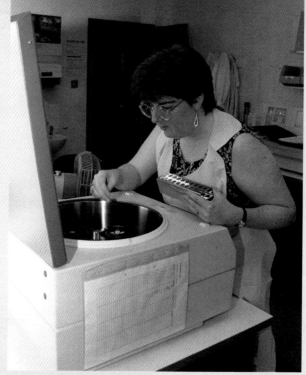

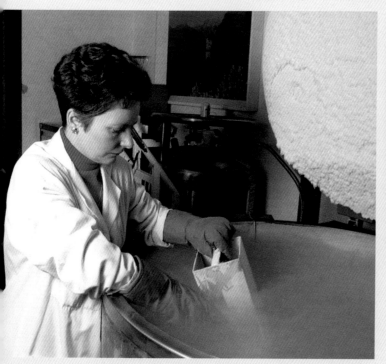

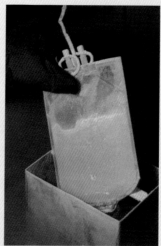

The Department of Haematology, like all the pathology departments, offers a full investigative service not only to the RUH but all the community hospitals and General Practitioners around Bath. (Above) MLSO Luci Clift is centrifuging samples for coagulation (clotting) investigations.

Bone marrow and peripheral stem cells harvested for use in patients with blood malignancies are stored deeply frozen in liquid nitrogen. (Left) Clinical Scientist Anne Smith is removing specimens from the liquid nitrogen tank.

(Right) The RUH receives weekly deliveries of liquid nitrogen.

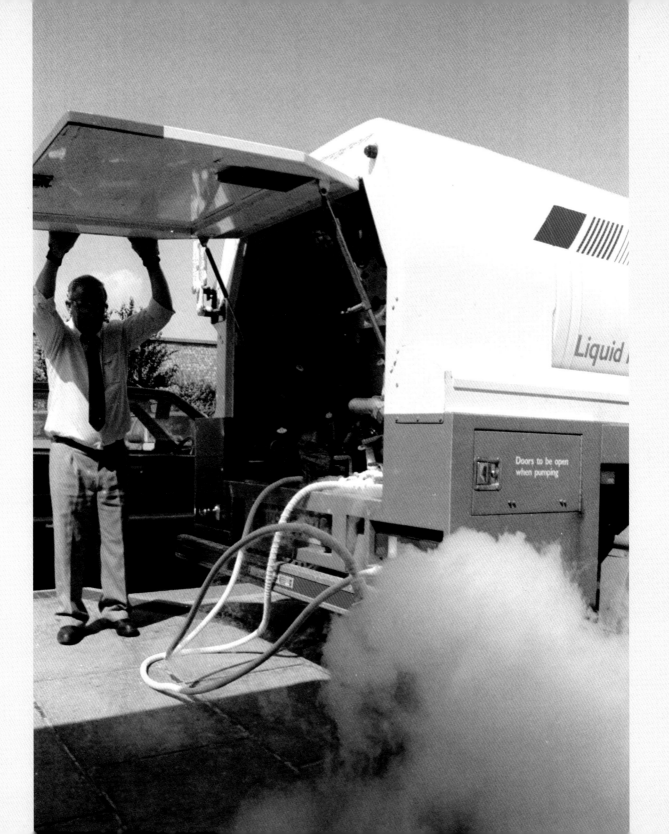

Catering for all...

The Catering Department was the first part of the hospital to undergo redevelopment during RUH 2001. The catering staff currently prepare approximately 9100 patient meals per week using, amongst other things, 4870 pints of milk, almost 1500 eggs and over 800 loaves of bread. Every week the catering staff also cook 2240 lbs of potatoes. As well as producing meals for patients, the Catering Department also provides food for staff at the RUH, supplies beverages and buffets for meetings, places food in vending machines and twice a week cooks for the residents of Fairfield House close to the hospital where food is delivered by Age Concern.

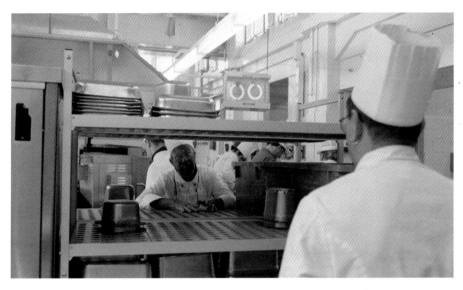

(Above) Chefs, Frank Rowsell and Robert Jarvis, discuss menu options.

(Below) Chef Melanie Pike preparing baked apples.

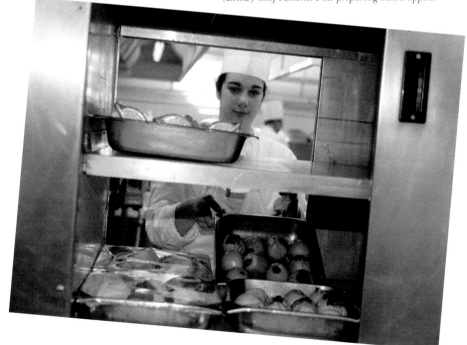

Cleanliness and hygiene are paramount within the department and Patrick Barror is seen here cleaning a steam boiling pan.

Paul Cox, Chef Supervisor.

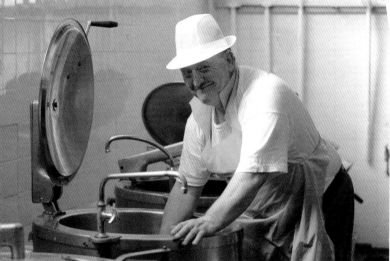

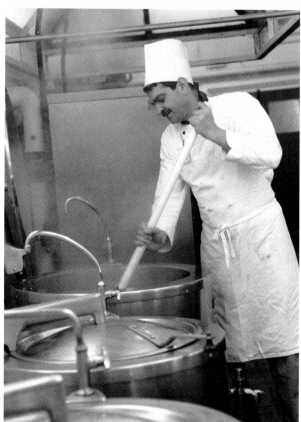

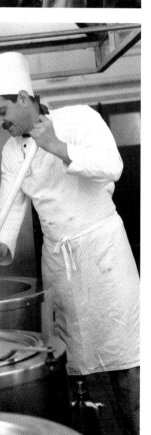

(Above) Tom Rowe and Dining Room Catering Assistant, Virginia Hill, are pictured in the wash-up area. This can get particularly hot and steamy, especially when there are lots of pans to be cleaned!

(Left) Chef Gerry Delauro.

87

Hysterectomy

Hysterectomy is the surgical removal of the uterus (womb). The operation may be performed through an incision in the lower abdomen or, in some circumstances, via the birth canal. Between 80 000 and 100 000 women undergo a hysterectomy each year in the UK.

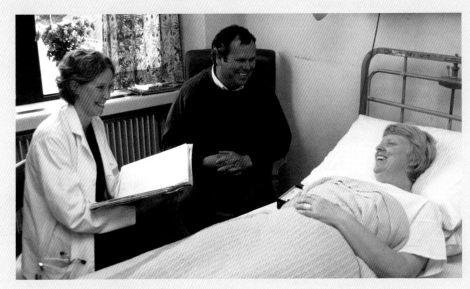

Belinda Lucas was admitted to the hospital on the morning of her planned hysterectomy. Her medical history was taken and the procedure explained to Mrs Lucas and her husband.

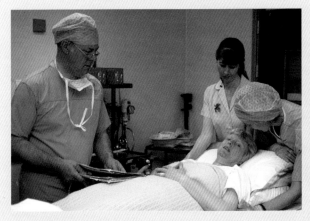

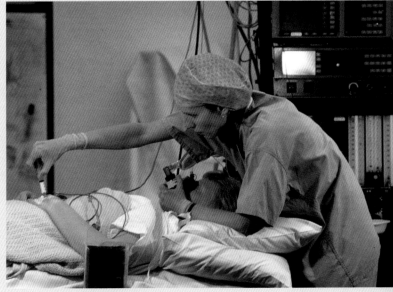

(Above) Mrs Lucas was taken to the operating theatre where her details were checked.

(Right) Consultant Anaesthetist Dr Alison Harries administered Mrs Lucas' anaesthetic into her vein whilst she breathed oxygen.

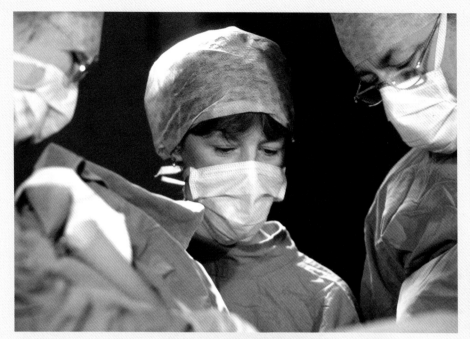

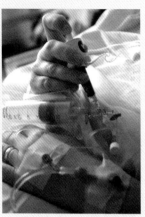

After the operation Dr Harries provided Mrs Lucas with a machine (PCA) to enable her to give herself repeated doses of a painkilling drug directly into her vein whenever she required.

(Above) Gynaecological Surgeons Mr Geoff Dunster and Miss Charlie Flemming and team carry out the operation.

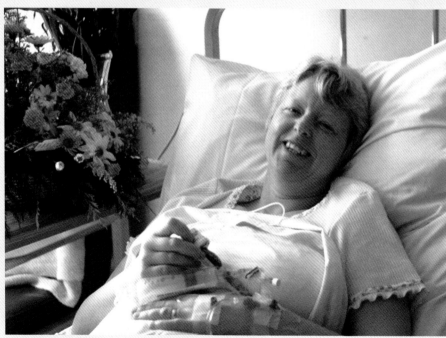

(Right) Within a few hours of the operation Mrs Lucas was back on the ward, keeping herself free from pain with her PCA.

And so to bed...

Like all acute hospitals, the RUH provides continuing care for its patients day and night, every day of the year. Patients are not admitted to the hospital electively out of hours but emergency admissions

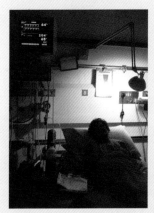

continue through the night. Some patients even require emergency surgery during the night or at weekends and the hospital has operating theatres and teams of theatre staff dedicated solely to the provision of emergency care.

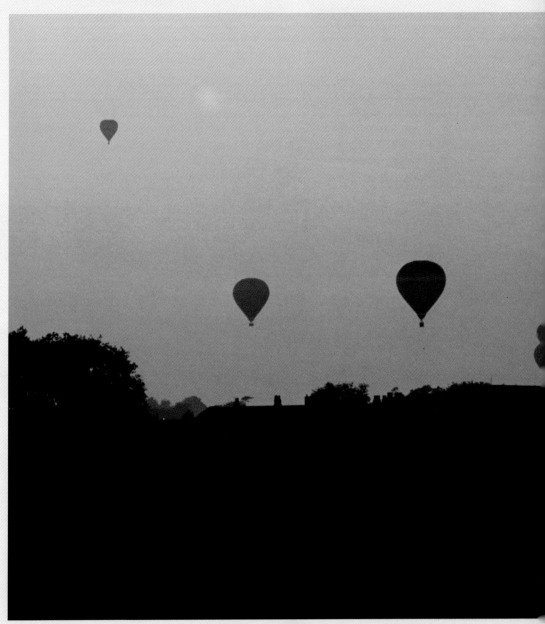

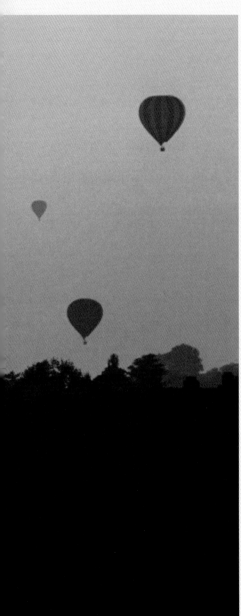

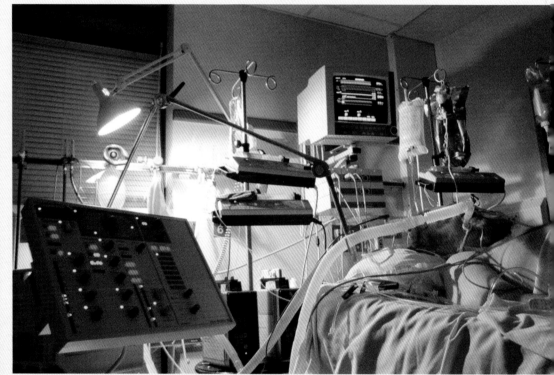

Our Hospital

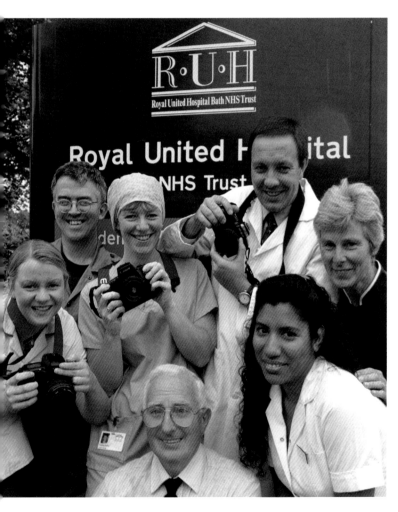

In 1996 the doctors and nurses of the Royal United Hospital developed a vision for how the RUH would serve its patients into the next century. This vision became known as RUH 2001. Construction work on the new part of the hospital commenced in 1997, exactly 250 years after the first hospital from which the RUH grew was opened in Bath. It became apparent that the RUH was about to enter a phase of change as great as any it had previously known. I felt that change on this scale needed to be recorded and that a book should be produced that reflected life at the RUH before the site redevelopment was completed. Furthermore, proceeds from sales of the book would directly contribute to the hospital's charitable fund. And so the idea for *Our Hospital* was born.

The most significant step I made towards making the idea a reality was to enlist the help and expertise of a colleague in the Department of Anaesthesia, Dr Mike Scott. As well as being an anaesthetist, Mike is also a semi-professional photographer with immense talent. There are many examples of Mike's art in *Our Hospital* including all the picture

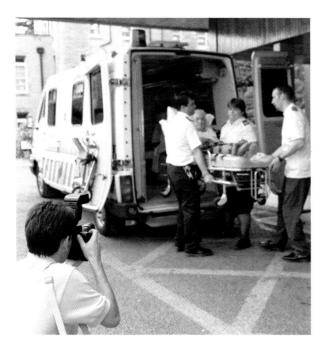

stories and the cover photographs. Mike gave freely of his time and skill and it is obvious that *Our Hospital* would look nothing like it does were it not for his generosity.

Next I needed a publisher to steer the project from concept to book. The obvious choice was BIOS Scientific Publishers Ltd in Oxford with whom I and others who work at the RUH already had a

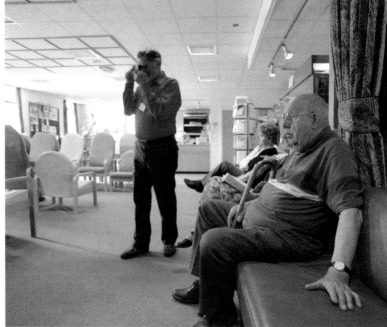

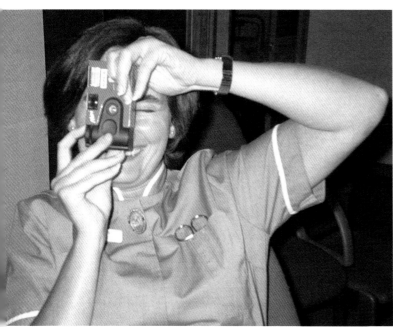

professional relationship. To his credit, Managing Director, Jonathan Ray, did not hesitate in agreeing to take on the project and to do so on a non-profit making basis. This meant that the charitable fund would benefit to a maximum from sales of the book. Lisa Mansell, Production Manager, joined the team and kept us focused throughout.

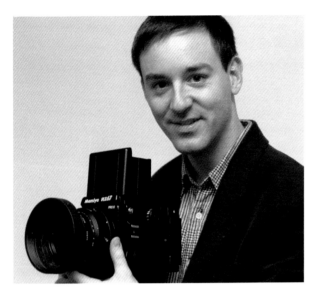

(Above) Dr Mike Scott.

(Below) Scanning a negative to create a digital image.

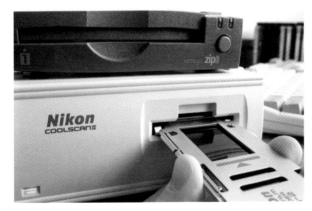

Bath is surrounded by a number of printing firms but we decided to start by approaching the best. Delightedly, Adrian Huett, Managing Director, and Tim Taylor, Marketing Manager, of the Butler & Tanner Group, agreed to produce *Our Hospital* as a charitable exercise from design through to print.

Our Hospital is a book about the RUH. It is full of photographs that reflect what being a patient, visitor, or working at the RUH felt like on one day in the Summer of 1997. It is not a comprehensive picture of all aspects of the RUH but simply a snap shot seen through the eyes (and lenses) of hundreds of people on one day. Anyone who was in the hospital on 7 July 1997 was given film for their camera, or a single use camera if they hadn't brought one with them, with which to take photos of their own perspective of that one day at the RUH. James Scott of Bayer Pharmaceuticals generously provided the rolls of film and the single use cameras and everyone got snapping. As well as these candid pictures being taken, two other highly skilled photographers, Chris Newton and Neil Eaton, joined Mike Scott on the day to encourage others in the use of their cameras and to take some of the more quirky shots themselves. Their help and support, given freely like all others involved in the book, is gratefully acknowledged.

This photographic frenzy resulted in almost 3000 pictures to be judged – thank you to all who took photographs or who starred in them, whether they made it to the final 200 in the book or not.

Then the work really started. The team gathered together to judge the photos and the final 200 were selected. Mike Scott painstakingly cleaned and scanned all the negatives and created digital images for the designers to use. Because we wanted all the photographs to be as high quality as possible, Mike also spent time

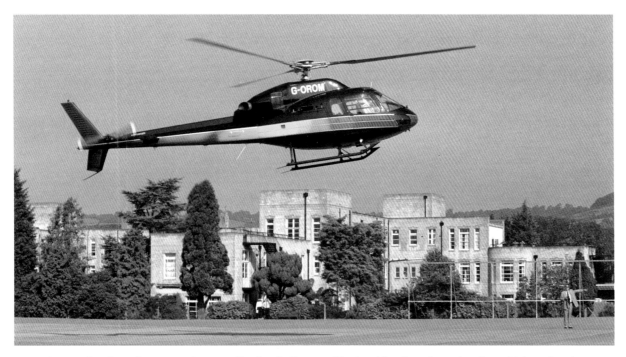

cropping and enhancing some images. Butler & Tanner Design/Section then developed ideas for the book layout whilst Lisa and I wrote the text to support some of the shots.

Since the original idea for the book grew from the plans to redevelop the hospital site, we really needed an aerial shot to put the site into perspective. After a couple of attempts spoiled by the weather, my great friend Colin Sanders finally landed his elegant twin-engined helicopter at the hospital and from G-OROM we got the shot of the site we wanted.

Throughout the project I was helped immensely by Corrine Porter at the RUH, in particular in co-ordinating the distribution and then collection and development of the films and cameras used on the day.

To all these people and the many others who helped produce *Our Hospital*, working on a non-profit basis so as to benefit the charitable fund as much as possible, I am deeply grateful. But most importantly I would like to thank you the reader on behalf of all the patients and staff of the Royal United Hospital, Bath for generously supporting our book.

Dr Tim Craft
Clinical Director of Anaesthesia, Theatres, Intensive Care, and Pain Services

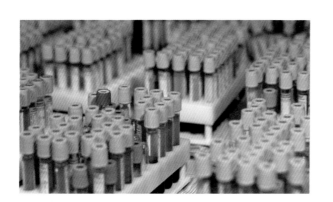

Acknowledgements

The generous contributions of the following are gratefully acknowledged:

Bayer Pharmaceuticals, Newbury

BIOS Scientific Publishers Ltd, Oxford

Butler & Tanner Group of Companies, Frome

Mike Scott Photography